The Labor Progress Handbook

Early Interventions to Prevent and Treat Dystocia

Second edition

Penny Simkin *BA, PT, CCE, CD (DONA)*
Seattle Midwifery School
Independent Practice of Childbirth Education and Labor Support

Ruth Ancheta *BA, ICCE, CD (DONA)*
Independent Practice of Childbirth Education and Labor Support

with

a chapter on assessing labor progress

Suzy Myers *LM, CPM, MPH*
Seattle Midwifery School
Seattle Home Maternity Service & Childbirth Center

Illustrated by **Shanna dela Cruz**

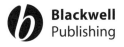

Blackwell
Publishing

© 2000, 2005 by Blackwell Publishing Ltd

Copyright for illustrations 1994, 1999 and 2004 and 2005 Ruth Ancheta

Editorial offices:
Blackwell Publishing Ltd, 9600 Garsington Road, Oxford OX4 2DQ, UK
 Tel: +44 (0)1865 776868
Blackwell Publishing Inc., 350 Main Street, Malden, MA 02148-5020, USA
 Tel: +1 781 388 8250
Blackwell Publishing Asia Pty Ltd, 550 Swanston Street, Carlton, Victoria 3053, Australia
 Tel: +61 (0)3 8359 1011

The right of the Author to be identified as the Author of this Work has been asserted in accordance with the Copyright, Designs and Patents Act 1988.

First published 2000 Blackwell Science Ltd
Second edition 2005

3   2008

Library of Congress Cataloging-in-Publication Data
Simkin, Penny, 1938–
   The labor progress handbook : early interventions to prevent and treat dystocia / Penny Simkin, Ruth Ancheta, with Suzy Myers; illustrated by Shanna dela Cruz. — 2nd ed.
   p. ; cm.
   Includes bibliographical references and index.
   ISBN-13: 978-1-4051-2217-7 (pbk. : alk. paper)
   ISBN-10: 1-4051-2217-X (pbk. : alk. paper)
   1. Labor (Obstetrics)—Complications—Prevention—Handbooks, manuals, etc. 2. Birth injuries—Prevention–Handbooks, manuals, etc.
   [DNLM: 1. Dystocia—prevention & control—Handbooks. 2. Birth Injuries—prevention & control—Handbooks. 3. Labor Complications—Handbooks. WQ 39 S589L 2005]
   I. Ancheta, Ruth. II. Myers, Suzy. III. Title.

RG701.S57 2005
618.5—dc22
                    2005005239

ISBN 13: 978-14051-2217-7
ISBN 10: 1-4051-2217-X

A catalogue record for this title is available from the British Library

Set in 9/11pt Plantin
by Graphicraft Limited, Hong Kong
Printed and bound in the USA
by Sheridan Books, Inc, Ann Arbor, MI

The publisher's policy is to use permanent paper from mills that operate a sustainable forestry policy, and which has been manufactured from pulp processed using acid-free and elementary chlorine-free practices. Furthermore, the publisher ensures that the text paper and cover board used have met acceptable environmental accreditation standards.

For further information on Blackwell Publishing, visit our website:
www.blackwellpublishing.com

Contents

Foreword to the second edition   xi
Foreword to the first edition   xv
Dedication   xvii
Acknowledgements   xviii

Chapter 1   Introduction   1

Some important differences in maternity care between the
   United States, the United Kingdom, and Canada   6
Notes on this book   6
Changes in this second edition   9
   Material on epidurals   9
Conclusion   9
References   10

Chapter 2   Dysfunctional Labor: General Considerations   11

What is normal labor?   11
What is dysfunctional labor?   13
Maintaining labor progress: prevention of dysfunctional
   labor   15
   A role for the fetus in regulating labor?   16
The psycho-emotional state of the woman: reducing
   maternal distress   16
   Psycho-emotional measures   18
   Physical comfort measures   20
   Physiological measures   21
Why focus on maternal position?   22
Monitoring the mobile woman's fetus   23
   Auscultation   24
   When electronic fetal monitoring is required:
      options to enhance maternal mobility   24

Continuous EFM	25
Intermittent EFM	27
Telemetry	28
Techniques to elicit stronger contractions	31
Conclusion	32
References	32

Chapter 3 Assessing Progress in Labor	**35**
Before labor begins	36
Malposition	36
Observing for clues to fetal position	38
Palpating for fetal position	39
Palpating using Leopold's maneuvers	40
Auscultating for fetal position	43
Belly mapping	44
Other assessments prior to labor	48
Assessments during labor	50
Position, attitude and descent of the fetus	50
Vaginal examinations: indications and timing	51
Performing a vaginal examination during labor	51
The vaginal exam, step by step	53
Assessing the cervix	54
Unusual cervical findings	55
The presenting part	56
The vagina and bony pelvis	64
Quality of contractions	64
Assessing the mother's condition	67
Assessing the fetus	69
How to perform intermittent auscultation	70
Reassuring signs of fetal well-being that can be assessed without EFM	72
Putting it all together	75
Assessing progress in first stage	75
Features of normal latent phase	76
Features of normal active phase	76
Assessing progress in second stage	77
Features of normal second stage	77
Conclusion	77
References	77

Chapter 4 Prolonged Pre-Labor and Latent First Stage **82**

Is it dystocia? 82
  When is a woman in labor? 83
  Preventing the occiput posterior (OP): measures to use before labor 84
  The woman who has hours of contractions without dilation 87
The six ways to progress in labor 87
Support measures for women who are at home in pre-labor and latent phase 89
Some reasons for excessive pain and duration of pre-labor or latent phase 91
  Iatrogenic factors 91
  Cervical factors 92
  Fetal factors 92
  Emotional factors 92
Troubleshooting measures for painful prolonged pre-labor or latent phase 93
Measures to alleviate painful irregular non-dilating contractions in pre-labor or latent phase 95
Synclitism and asynclitism 95
Conclusion 101
References 101

Chapter 5 Prolonged Active Phase of Labor **103**

What is prolonged active labor? 104
Characteristics of prolonged active labor 105
Possible causes of prolonged active labor 106
  Fetal and feto-pelvic factors 108
  Why fetal malpositions delay labor progress 110
  Artificial rupture of the membranes (AROM) with a malpositioned fetus 111
  Specific measures to address and correct problems associated with malposition, cephalo-pelvic disproportion and macrosomia 112
Maternal positions and movements for suspected malposition, cephalo-pelvic disproportion, or macrosomia in active labor 112

Forward-leaning positions 114
Side-lying positions 116
Asymmetrical positions and movements 118
Abdominal lifting 120
An uncontrollable premature urge to push 120
If contractions are inadequate 123
Immobility 123
Medication 125
Dehydration 126
Exhaustion 126
Uterine lactic acidosis as a cause of inadequate
contractions 127
When the cause of inadequate contractions is unknown 128
If there is a persistent cervical lip or a swollen cervix 131
Position changes to reduce an anterior lip or a swollen
cervix 132
Other methods 132
Manual reduction of a persistent cervical lip 133
If emotional dystocia is suspected 134
Assessing the woman's coping 134
Indicators of emotional dystocia during active labor 136
Predisposing factors for emotional dystocia 136
Helping the woman state her fears 137
How to help a laboring woman in distress 138
Special needs of childhood abuse survivors 140
Incompatibility or poor relationship with staff 141
If the source of the woman's anxiety cannot be identified 142
Conclusion 142
References 143

Chapter 6   Prolonged Second Stage of Labor 146

Definitions of the second stage of labor 146
The phases of the second stage 147
The latent phase of the second stage 147
The active phase of the second stage 150
If the woman has an epidural 156
How long an active phase of second stage is too long? 161
Possible etiologies and solutions for second-stage
dystocia 162

Positions and other strategies for suspected occiput
  posterior (OP) or persistent occiput transverse (OT)
  fetuses   162
Why not the dorsal position?   162
Differentiating between pushing positions and birth
  positions   165
Manual interventions to reposition the OP fetus   174
Early interventions for suspected persistent asynclitism   174
If cephalo-pelvic disproportion (CPD) or macrosomia is
  suspected   177
Positions for 'possible CPD' in second stage   178
Shoulder dystocia   188
If contractions are inadequate   188
If emotional dystocia is suspected   188
Conclusion   192
References   193

Chapter 7   The Labor Progress Toolkit: Part 1.
            Maternal Positions and Movements   **196**

Maternal positions   197
  Side-lying positions   198
  The 'side-lying lunge'   202
  Semi-sitting   203
  Sitting upright   205
  Sitting leaning forward with support   207
  Standing, leaning forward   208
  Kneeling, leaning forward with support   210
  Hands and knees   212
  Open knee–chest position   213
  Closed knee–chest position   215
  Asymmetrical upright (standing, kneeling, sitting)
    positions   216
  Squatting   218
  Supported squatting positions   220
  Half squatting, lunging and swaying   222
  Lap squatting   224
  Exaggerated lithotomy (McRoberts' position)   226
  Supine   228
  Rope pull   229

Maternal movements	231
Pelvic rocking (also called pelvic tilt) and other movements of the pelvis	231
The lunge	233
Walking or stair climbing	235
Slow dancing	236
Abdominal stroking	238
Abdominal lifting	239
The pelvic press	241
Other rhythmic movements	243
References	244

Chapter 8   The Labor Progress Toolkit: Part 2. Comfort Measures   **246**

General guidelines for comfort during a slow labor	247
Non-pharmacological physical comfort measures	248
Heat	248
Cold	250
Hydrotherapy	252
Touch and massage	257
Acupressure	259
Acupuncture	260
Continuous labor support from a doula, nurse, or midwife	262
Psychosocial comfort measures	265
Assessing the woman's emotional state	265
Techniques and devices to reduce back pain	268
Counter-pressure	268
The double hip squeeze	269
The knee press	272
Cold and heat	273
Hydrotherapy	275
Movement	276
Birth ball	277
Transcutaneous electrical nerve stimulation (TENS)	278
Intradermal sterile water injections for back pain (ID water blocks)	281
Breathing for relaxation and a sense of mastery	283

Bearing-down techniques for the second stage   285
Conclusion   287
References   287

Epidural Index   290
Index   291

Foreword to the second edition

In Canada, where we pride ourselves on having an integrated system of maternity care, where obstetricians, family doctors, nurses, and midwives work collaboratively, a recent national study nevertheless reported that three out of four women receive one or more major interventions in labor. How can this be? Could it be because we have forgotten how to look after women in labor?

The second edition of this thoughtful and practical book will be a gift to the full range of practitioners and trainees from the sister disciplines of obstetrics and gynecology, family practice, midwifery and nursing. It is a skillful blend of classical obstetrical teaching, quoting liberally from conventional textbooks and scientific literature, to 'new' information gleaned from the long experience of midwives.

Generations of medical students have learned a huge amount about the pathology of childbirth, with the result that they tend to fear labor and have learned to intervene with the 'big guns', like oxytocin augmentation and various forms of expedited birth. We learned as students that childbirth could be reduced to a little plumbing: the 'three Ps'. And if we regurgitated this in an exam, we received a sure pass.

(1) The *Passage* or pelvis: size, shape, angles.
(2) The *Power* or strength of contractions.
(3) The *Passenger* or fetus, meaning principally the size of fetal head but also position and attitude.

Unfortunately, while plumbing is important in childbirth and in life (especially for those of us in advancing years), there is so much more to labor and life. Responding to the complexity and simplicity of labor so well described in this book, some of us have invented another 'seven Ps', and I was pleased to find that many of them have been enumerated by the authors:

(4) The *Person* – the woman: her beliefs, preparation, knowledge and 'capacity' for doing the work of labor and birth.

(5) The *Partner* – how the woman is supported and the partner's knowledge, beliefs and preparation for the labor.

(6) The *People* – the 'entourage' – others who may be involved in the pregnancy, labor and birth process, and who are working with the woman. The entourage also have their beliefs, preparation, and knowledge of the process, and this interacts positively or negatively with those of the woman and her partner.

(7) The *Pain* – the influence and experience of pain and the socio-cultural beliefs of the woman and her support system and her personal psychological environment. All this influences the woman's capacity for coping with labor and birth. Clearly pain interpretation and pain control impacts the progress of labor.

(8) The *Professionals* – the manner in which all members of the health care team support, inform and collaborate in care and information-sharing with the woman and her partner and support people, significantly influences the woman's response to the labor and birth process.

(9) The *Passion* – the journey of pregnancy, labor and birth, is one that is special and unique for all women. It is crucial for all involved in the care of women to recognize and honor this passion and allow this concept to guide us in our practice as we appreciate and guard the intimacy of this life-changing experience. And we need to control our anxiety and need for perfection so that the woman can fully experience the passion even when the birth is complex and requires considerable help from us.

(10) The *Politics* – You know it's true!

This book focuses on these concepts, while providing concrete information to help us facilitate the natural processes that are ready to be released, if we but give them time.

How refreshing to find a book that teaches how to stay out of trouble, how to prevent dysfunctional labors (and even to do so well before labor occurs) during prenatal care. It is liberating to have information on how to shift a fetus from an unfavorable to a favorable position, rather than waiting pessimistically to see an antenatal fetal malposition turn into an intrapartum OT or OP. New learners will benefit from the detailed descriptions of asynclitism and how to diagnose and treat it, as well as excellent descriptions of how to diagnose a flexed or extended head.

I have seen Penny teach these techniques in workshops for maternity caregivers, and seen the 'Aha!' experience that results in the statement, 'I can't wait to try these techniques in my next clinic or labor'. And now the information is available in accessible form to share with trainees and the women themselves. Thus, this book complements and augments the materials conventionally taught to medical students and specialist trainees. It will empower them with information that they can use in the labor suite. It will make them feel useful.

Epidural analgesia: the new reality. Who can argue with good pain relief? But at what price? And do women know, and have they been taught the full picture? The Cochrane Collaboration clearly demonstrates that it increases the length of the first and second stages of labor, increases the use of instrumentation and leads to excess perineal trauma. And while Cochrane reports no increase in cesarean section, most of us know that to be untrue. When used early and often (not the conditions of the major new trials in Cochrane)[1], epidural analgesia usually requires oxytocin augmentation (which is generally given in low dose regimes). Epidural analgesia clearly increases the frequency of cesarean section.

Therefore, I was particularly impressed with the way that the authors explained the influence of epidural analgesia on the course of labor. In fact, epidural analgesia is now so pervasive that we have forgotten how the entire shape of labor has been altered by its availability and omnipresence. Not to overstate the issue, there are places in North America and elsewhere where the staff either do not know or have forgotten how to look after women who do not have an epidural. Unfortunately, it is this sad situation that makes it so necessary to describe how epidural analgesia alters labor and what techniques are needed to assist women who have an epidural. The authors have therefore elaborated on this new reality and provided the cautions and tools to assist caregivers do their best to let labor unfold in the presence of an epidural.

This little text, which will fit nicely in a back pocket or 'lab coat', provides practical diagrams of normal and abnormal fetal positions that can be identified well before labor, and more importantly, corrected, so as to lessen the malpositions of labor that unleash the 'cascade' of interventions that characterize the experience of so many women having their first babies. It will take much to turn society back from thinking of childbirth as an accident waiting to happen and to help women realize their power and competence, but the authors have given us a tool to help in that process, to help us keep normal birth normal. I am grateful that this book is available and entering its second edition.

Michael C. Klein   *MD, CCFP,*
FAAP(Neonatal-Perinatal), FCFP, ABFP
Emeritus Professor of Family Practice and Pediatrics
University of British Columbia

REFERENCE

1. Howell, C. (2000) Epidural versus non-epidural analgesia for pain relief in labour. Cochrane Database Systematic Review, Issue 3. Art. No: CD000331. DOI: 10.1002/14651858.CD000331.

Foreword to the first edition

At last, a book that offers practical advice for nurses and midwives who wish to help to prevent and treat dysfunctional labor! Penny Simkin and Ruth Ancheta have done a superb job of interweaving the clinical wisdom of observant, expert practitioners with the best available research evidence about what helps and does not help women during labor.

I wish this book had been available a long time ago. In the early 1970s when I was a novice labor and delivery nurse, I observed a common but puzzling problem. In those days we subjected women to an admission routine that included a variety of very unpleasant procedures. (Thankfully the worst of these procedures – perineal shaves, enemas, and rectal exams – have since been recognized as useless or harmful and have been eliminated from common practice.) Part of the admission routine involved assessment of the quality and strength of contractions. When I inquired about the contractions, I was often told, 'My contractions were frequent and strong at home, but they seem to have gotten a lot weaker and further apart since I arrived.'

I would reply, 'Do not worry, this happens a lot. After we finish the admission procedures and you are settled in here, your labor will probably get going again.'

Why did I say this? I believed it. I had observed it often and had overheard experienced colleagues reassure their patients in this way. At some intuitive level I felt the decrease in labor intensity was caused by the woman's reaction to the stress of the hospital admission routine. But at the time almost nothing had been written about the role of stress hormones on uterine function, nor about the relationships between maternal anxiety, environmental influences, stress hormones, and labor complications. And the randomized controlled trials showing the substantial benefits of labor support had not even been conducted yet[1].

What about the instances in which labor did not return spontaneously to the strong, regular pattern that had been occurring prior to admission? Our repertoire of nursing interventions was limited primarily to advising the woman either to ambulate or to rest and wait. (Currently, in some settings the options may be even fewer, with ambulation restricted by the routine use of electronic fetal monitors.) These women frequently ended up with a cascade of medical interventions – IV oxytocin, amniotomy, epidural analgesia, and forceps or cesarean delivery.

I now believe that there is much more I could have done to prevent or treat the problem of dysfunctional labor. Penny Simkin and Ruth Ancheta have described how 'emotional dystocia' and stressful environmental influences may lead to complications, and they offer simple but potentially powerful nursing measures to ameliorate these problems. They have also persuaded me that many instances of dystocia or prolonged labor may be caused by subtle malpositions of the fetal head, potentially correctable with simple positioning techniques.

I can only imagine how much more effective I would have been if this book had been available when I was a labor and delivery nurse. As a researcher, I am inspired to study these simple but potentially very powerful labor support techniques. Dystocia or dysfunctional labor is the most common reason for primary cesarean delivery. Given the high rates of cesarean delivery in North America and the UK, and the limitations and risks of medical treatments for dystocia, it seems long overdue that nurses and midwives take an active role in preventing and treating this common clinical problem. This book contains a wealth of information about and practical suggestions for preventing and correcting dysfunctional labor. It should be required reading for all who care for women in labor, and a reference text in every labor and birthing unit.

Ellen D. Hodnett *RN, PhD*
Professor and Heather M. Reisman Chair
Perinatal Nursing Research
University of Toronto

REFERENCE

1. Hodnett, E. (1998) Support from caregivers during childbirth (Cochrane Review). In: *The Cochrane Library*, Issue 3. Update Software, Oxford.

Dedication

We dedicate this book to childbearing women and their caregivers in the hope that some of our suggestions will reduce the likelihood of cesarean delivery for dystocia; also to the wise, patient and observant midwives, nurses, doulas, family doctors and obstetricians whose actions and writings have inspired and taught us.

Acknowledgements

We have been helped in writing this book by many wonderful people, especially:

- Sally Avenson, Fredrik Broekhuizen, Roberta Gehrke, Lynn Diulio, Mary Mazul, Jean Sutton, Karen Hillegas, Barbara Kalmen, Karen Kohls, Ann Krigbaum, and Karen Lupa for their helpful suggestions
- John Carroll, Alicia Huntley, Shauna Leinbach, Jenn McAllister, Sara Wickham, and Lisa Hanson for reviewing the text and giving us useful feedback
- Diony Young, for her assistance and support
- Anne Frye, midwife and author of *Holistic Midwifery*, for her stimulating conversation and generous sharing of ideas
- Shanna dela Cruz, our dedicated and meticulous illustrator
- Sharon Simkin, who provided the cover photo
- Shona Simkin and Avery Tipper, shown on the book cover
- The dozens of women and men who posed for our illustrations, especially Carissa and Zsolt Farkas, Robin Block, Asela Calhoun, Vic dela Cruz, Helen Vella Dentice, Maureen Wahhab, Bob Meidl, and Lori Meidl Zahorodney, and staff members of Waukesha Memorial Hospital, Aurora Sinai Hospital, and St. Mary's Hospital of Milwaukee, Wisconsin, USA
- Celia Bannenberg, for permission to redraw the DeBy birthing stool
- PrePak Products for permission to show The Rope (the "birthing rope")
- Gail Tully, author of "*Spinning Babies: Childbirth Made Easier With Fetal Positioning*," for contributing her material for the section on "Belly Mapping" in Chapter 3
- Lesley James, Jan Dowers, Tracy Sachjen, and Heather Snookal, who provided support and assistance with word processing, communication, and other ways of making our lives easier
- Last but not least, our families who have helped us in countless ways as we devoted ourselves to this larger than expected task

Chapter 1

Introduction

Some important differences in maternity care between the United States, the United Kingdom, and Canada, 6
Notes on this book, 6
Changes in this second edition, 9
Material on epidurals, 9
Conclusion, 9
References, 10

Labor dystocia, dysfunctional labor, failure to progress, arrest of labor, arrested descent – all these terms refer to slow or no progress in labor, which is one of the most vexing, complex and unpredictable complications of labor. Labor dystocia is the most common medical indication for primary cesarean sections. In countries where rates of vaginal births after previous cesareans (VBAC) are low (for example, in the United States in 2003 the VBAC rate was less than 11%[1], having dropped from a high of almost 30% in 1996[2]), dystocia also contributes indirectly to the number of repeat cesareans. The American College of Obstetricians and Gynecologists estimates that 60% of all cesareans in the USA are attributable to the diagnosis of dystocia[3]. With a primary cesarean rate of 19.1%, and a total rate of 27.6%[1] (or more than 1 million cesareans) in 2003, it is clear that prevention of dystocia would not only reduce the number of costly and risky obstetric interventions, including cesareans, but it would also spare some women the feelings of discouragement and disappointment that often accompany a prolonged or complicated birth.

1

The possible causes of labor dystocia are numerous. Some are intrinsic:

- The *powers* (the uterine contractions)
- The *passage* (size, shape, and joint mobility of the pelvis, and the stretch and resilience of the vaginal canal)
- The *passenger* (size and shape of fetal head, fetal presentation and position)
- The *pain* (and the woman's ability to cope with it)
- The *psyche* (anxiety, emotional state of the woman)

Others are extrinsic:

- *Environment* (the feelings of physical and emotional safety generated by the setting and the people surrounding the woman)
- *Ethno-cultural* factors (the degree of sensitivity and respect for the woman's culture-based needs and preferences)
- *Hospital or caregiver policies* (how flexible, family- or woman-centered, how evidence-based)
- *Psycho-emotional care* (the priority given to non-medical aspects of the childbirth experience)

Please see Michael Klein's Foreword to this edition for his discussion of factors influencing labor progress.

This book focuses on prevention, differential diagnosis, and early interventions to use with dysfunctional labor. The emphasis is on relatively simple and sensible care measures or interventions designed to help maintain normal labor progress and to manage and correct minor complications before they become serious enough to require major interventions. We believe this approach is consistent with worldwide efforts, including those of the World Health Organization, to reserve the use of medical interventions for situations in which they are needed: 'The aim of the care [in normal birth] is to achieve a healthy mother and baby with the least possible level of intervention that is compatible with safety[4].'

The suggestions in this book are based on the following premises:

- Progress may slow or stop for any of a number of reasons at any time in labor – pre-labor, early labor, active labor, or during the second or third stage.
- The timing of the delay is an important consideration when establishing cause and selecting interventions.

- Sometimes several causal factors may occur at one time.
- Caregivers and others are often able to enhance or maintain labor progress with simple non-surgical, non-pharmacological physical and psychological interventions. Such interventions have the following advantages:
  - compared to most obstetric interventions for dystocia, they carry less risk of harm or undesirable side effects to mother or baby
  - they treat the woman as the key to the solution, not the key to the problem
  - they build or strengthen the cooperation between the woman, her support people (loved ones, doula), and caregivers
  - they reduce the need for riskier, costlier, more complex interventions
  - they may increase the woman's emotional satisfaction with her experience of birth

- The choice of solutions depends on the causal factors, if known, but trial and error is sometimes necessary when the cause is unclear. The greatest drawbacks are that the woman may not want to try these interventions, they sometimes take time, or they may not correct the problem.
- Time is usually an ally, not an enemy. With time, many problems in labor progress are resolved. In the absence of clear medical or psychological contraindications, patience, reassurance and low or no risk interventions may constitute the most appropriate course of management.
- The caregiver may use the following in determining the cause of the problem(s):
  - *objective observations*: woman's vital signs; fetal heart rate patterns; fetal presentation, position and size; cervical assessments; assessments of contraction strength, frequency, and duration; membrane status; and time
  - *subjective observations*: woman's affect, description of pain, level of fatigue
  - *direct questions* of the woman and *collaboration* with her in decisions regarding treatment:

    'What was going through your mind during that contraction?'
    'Please describe your pain.'
    'Why do you think labor has slowed down?'
    'Which options for treatment do you prefer?'

1

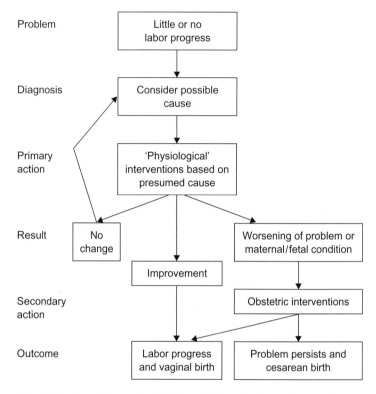

Problem — Little or no labor progress

Diagnosis — Consider possible cause

Primary action — 'Physiological' interventions based on presumed cause

Result — No change | Improvement | Worsening of problem or maternal/fetal condition

Secondary action — Obstetric interventions

Outcome — Labor progress and vaginal birth | Problem persists and cesarean birth

Chart 1.1   Care Plan for the Problem, 'Little or No Labor Progress'.

- Once the probable cause and the woman's perceptions and views are determined, appropriate primary interventions are instituted and labor progress is further observed. The problem may be solved with no further interventions.
- If the primary interventions are medically contraindicated or if they are unsuccessful, then obstetrical interventions are instituted under the guidance of the doctor or midwife.

Chart 1.1 illustrates the approach described in this book. Other similar flowcharts appear throughout this book to illustrate the application of this approach to a variety of causes of dysfunctional labor.

Many of the interventions described in this book are derived from the medical, midwifery, nursing, and childbirth education literature. Others come from the psychology, sociology, and anthropology literature. We have provided references for these, when available. Some suggestions have come from the extensive experience of nurses, midwives, doctors, and doulas (labor support providers). Many are applications of physical therapy principles and practices. Some items fall into the category of 'shared wisdom', where the original sources are unknown. We apologize if we neglect to mention the originator of an idea that has become widespread enough to fall into this category. Finally, some ideas originated with one or both of the authors who have used them successfully in their work with laboring women.

With today's emphasis on evidence-based practice, many rather entrenched maternity care customs are falling out of favor because they have been proven ineffective or harmful. Such routine practices as enemas, pubic shaving, continuous electronic fetal monitoring without access to fetal scalp blood sampling, the use of maternal supine and lithotomy positions in the second stage of labor, and routine episiotomy are some examples of forms of care that became widespread before they were scientifically evaluated. Then, once well-controlled trials of safety and effectiveness had been performed and the results combined in meta-analyses, these common practices were found to be ineffective and to increase risks[5].

Where possible, we will base our suggestions on such scientific evidence and will cite appropriate references. However, numerous simple and apparently risk-free practices have never been scientifically studied. Some of these are based on an understanding of the emotional and physiological processes taking place during childbirth. Others are applications of anatomy, kinesiology, and body mechanics to enhance the relationships between such separate but interdependent forces as pelvic shape, maternal posture, fetal position and station, uterine activity, and the force of gravity. Still others are based on a recognition of the importance of each laboring woman's personal and cultural values.

Some of the strategies suggested in this book will lend themselves well to randomized controlled trials, while others may not. Perhaps readers will gather ideas for scientific study as they read this book and apply its suggestions.

1

SOME IMPORTANT DIFFERENCES IN MATERNITY CARE BETWEEN THE UNITED STATES, THE UNITED KINGDOM, AND CANADA

This book is being published simultaneously in North America and the United Kingdom, where the approaches to maternity care are quite different from one another. It may surprise the reader to discover some of those differences, and it may also be interesting to learn that practices that are considered essential for safety in one country are considered ineffective or archaic in another. We hope that one effect of our book will be to encourage a willingness to reconsider practices that are either entrenched or avoided in one's own workplace.

Table 1.1 compares some basic features of maternity care between the United States, Canada, and the United Kingdom. Because of such differences in maternity care as those listed in Table 1.1, the willingness to introduce new practices and the power to do so will vary among caregivers in different countries. We hope our readers will begin to utilize the simplest, most innocuous measures immediately, and to educate themselves and change policies where necessary.

NOTES ON THIS BOOK

This book is directed toward midwives, nurses, and doctors who want to support and enhance the physiological process of labor, with the objective of avoiding complex, costly, more risky interventions. It will also be helpful for students in obstetrics, midwifery, and maternity nursing, for childbirth educators who can teach many of these techniques to expectant parents, and for doulas (trained labor support providers). The chapters are arranged chronologically according to the phases and stages of labor.

Because a particular maternal position or movement is useful for the same problem during more than one phase of labor, we have included illustrations of these positions in more than one chapter. This will allow the reader to find position ideas at a glance when working with a laboring woman. Complete descriptions of all the positions, movements, and other measures can be found in the Toolkit, Chapters 7 and 8.

The term 'caregiver' is used to refer to any of the people mentioned above who are providing care and support for the woman in labor.

Table 1.1 Comparison of maternity care in the United States, Canada, and the United Kingdom.

Feature	United States	Canada	United Kingdom
Primary maternity caregivers	Obstetricians for approximately 90% of women; midwives and family physicians for 10%. Maternity nurses provide most of the care during labor in the hospital, with the obstetrician managing any problems and the delivery.	Family physicians, with obstetricians and autonomous midwives now increasing in numbers. As in the USA, nurses provide most in-hospital care.	Mostly midwives, some general practitioners, with obstetricians caring for women with complications. There are no maternity nurses. Midwives provide all intrapartum care and conduct most deliveries.
Autonomy and independence of caregiver	Great variation in preferred routines among independent physicians. Nursing care varies according to the orders of each physician. Insurance providers and health maintenance organizations now increasingly limit those physicians' practices that are not cost effective.	Government limits payment for some interventions, and regulates numbers of doctors and hospitals, giving doctors less autonomy than in the USA.	Midwives have little autonomy, and practice according to the policies of their institutions. Those policies are established by authorities in maternity care and by the government.
Participation by childbearing women in decision-making	'Informed consent' is the law, though most women (except assertive women with strong opinions) expect the obstetrician to make decisions and most obstetricians prefer that style of practice. Most midwives and family physicians share decision making with the woman.	Similar to the USA.	'Informed choice' and 'woman-centered care' are now standards of care, and extensive efforts are being made by government and childbirth activists to ensure that women are well informed for their role as partners in decision making.

Continuity of caregiver throughout the childbearing year	Not considered cost effective, feasible, or desirable by policy-makers in health care. Rarely available except for out of hospital births, though to many women it is a highly desirable option. Some assertive women try to obtain continuity of care through birth plans and doulas, and by verbalizing their concerns to each professional involved in their care.	Small group practices of family physicians or midwives are available in many parts of Canada. Continuity of caregiver during pregnancy and post partum is more likely than in the USA, although maternity nurses provide most care in labor.	Considered a very important feature of woman-centered care, programs ensuring continuity of caregiver are beginning to replace the old system of different midwives for pre- and postnatal and intrapartum care.
Influence of scientific evidence on maternity practices	Highly variable, but customs, peer practices, opinions, and prior experience of the practitioner and fear of litigation are more powerful influences. Some medical, nursing, and midwifery schools now teach and follow principles of evidence-based practice.	Leaders in obstetrics, family medicine, midwifery, and nursing are actively engaged in scientific evaluation of numerous unproved clinical practices. The national professional societies of midwives, family physicians, obstetricians, and nurses promote evidence-based practice.	Same as Canada, except that midwives are also actively involved in research. There is widespread acceptance of a scientific approach to maternity care, where possible.
Influence of fear of malpractice litigation on maternity practices	The likelihood of doctors being sued for malpractice is high, and malpractice insurance premiums are extremely expensive, which has driven up the costs of maternity care. In addition, insurers advise on how to reduce the likelihood of lawsuits. Such advice is not based on science, safety or effectiveness, but on risks of being sued.	Trends similar to the USA, although to a much lesser degree. Fear of litigation has less impact on care than scientific findings, costs, customs and other factors.	Similar to Canada.

CHANGES IN THIS SECOND EDITION

Besides updating the information, suggestions, illustrations, and references throughout this edition, we have asked Suzy Myers, Licensed Midwife in Washington State, USA, to provide a new chapter on 'Assessing Progress in Labor'. She offers scientific evidence and lessons learned empirically over 25 years of attending births in free-standing birth centers and at home, along with many years of teaching midwives at Seattle Midwifery School. Her chapter offers techniques and practical tips that are not taught in many schools of medicine, midwifery, and nursing. For beginners, this chapter will serve as a text. For experienced professionals, this chapter will provide some useful additions to their already considerable repertoire. The innovative concept of 'belly mapping', developed by a Minnesota midwife and artist, Gail Tully, is also presented in this chapter, as a fully integrated approach to determine fetal position. This model uses clues gleaned from the clinical skills of the caregiver and the woman's observations of her fetus' movements. Gail Tully supplied the content and drawings for the 'belly mapping' segment of the chapter.

Material on epidurals

In acknowledgement of the widespread use of epidural analgesia, we address the needs of readers who work extensively with women who have epidurals and are unable to use many of the measures shown in this book. Labors with epidural analgesia are frequently accompanied by slow progress and the use of synthetic oxytocin. For this reason, to help readers quickly identify those measures that can be used with women with epidurals to correct fetal malpositions and to aid progress, we have prepared a special 'Epidural Index' to indicate locations of illustrations and text that are useful for women with epidurals.

CONCLUSION

The current emphasis in obstetrics is to find better ways to treat dystocia once it occurs. Little emphasis is placed on prevention, which is the focus of this book.

   To our knowledge, this is the first book that compiles labor progress strategies that can be used by a variety of caregivers in a variety of locations. Most of the strategies described can be used for births occurring in hospitals, at home, and in free-standing birth centers.

We hope this book will make your work more effective and more rewarding. Your knowledge of appropriate early interventions may spare many women from long, discouraging, or exhausting labors, reduce the need for major interventions, and contribute to safer and more satisfying outcomes. The women may not recognize specific things you have done for them, but they will appreciate and always remember your attentiveness, expertise, and support, which contribute so much to satisfaction[6] and positive long-term memories of their childbirths[7].

We wish you much success and fulfillment in your important work.

REFERENCES

1. Hamilton, B., Martin, J. & Sutton, P. (2004) Births: Preliminary Data for 2003. *National Vital Statistics Report*, **53**, 1–18. National Center for Health Statistics, Hyattesville, Maryland.
2. Center for Disease Control/National Center for Health Statistics (1998) *Monthly Vital Statistics Report, 1995–1998*. CDC, Atlanta.
3. American College of Obstetricians and Gynecologists (ACOG). (2003) Dystocia and augmentation of labor. ACOG Practice Bulletin, Number 49. *Obstetrics and Gynecology*, **102**, 1445–54.
4. WHO (1996) Chapter 1 Care in normal birth: a practical guide. In: *Safe Motherhood*. World Health Organization, Geneva.
5. Enkin, M., Keirse, M.J.N.C., Neilson, J., *et al.* (2000) *A Guide to Effective Care in Pregnancy and Childbirth*, 3rd edn. Oxford University Press, Oxford.
6. Hodnett, E. (2002) Pain and women's satisfaction with the experience of childbirth: a systematic review. *American Journal of Obstetrics and Gynecology*, **186** (5), s160–72.
7. Simkin, P. (1990) Just another day in a woman's life? Women's long-term perceptions of their first birth experience. Part I. *Birth*, **18** (4), 203–10.

Chapter 2

Dysfunctional Labor: General Considerations

What is normal labor? 11
What is dysfunctional labor?, 13
Maintaining labor progress: prevention of dysfunctional labor, 15
A role for the fetus in regulating labor? 16
The psycho-emotional state of the woman: reducing maternal distress, 16
Psycho-emotional measures, 18
Physical comfort measures, 20
Physiological measures, 21
Why focus on maternal position? 22
Monitoring the mobile woman's fetus, 23
Auscultation, 24
When electronic fetal monitoring is required: options to enhance maternal mobility, 24
Continuous EFM, 25
Intermittent EFM, 27
Telemetry, 28
Techniques to elicit stronger contractions, 31
Conclusion, 32
References, 32

WHAT IS NORMAL LABOR?

Normal labors may be long or short. They may very painful or hardly painful. They may occur after a high risk or low risk pregnancy. They may result in the birth of a small or a large baby. They may take place within or outside the hospital.

Despite these variations, all such labors, if they meet the following criteria, would be considered normal by the World Health

Organization (WHO)[1], which defines normal labor as having the following features:

- Spontaneous onset of labor between 37 and 42 completed weeks of pregnancy
- Low risk at the start, and remaining so throughout labor and delivery
- Spontaneous birth of an infant in the vertex presentation
- Mother and baby in good condition after birth

It is often stated that one can diagnose normal labor only in retrospect, leading many to conclude that it is preferable to treat all labors as high-risk, even though WHO estimates that 'between 70 and 80% of all pregnant women may be considered as low-risk at the start of labour'[1]. In recognition of the large expense, intensive training and actual risks inherent in treating all labors as high-risk, WHO states, 'In normal birth there should be a valid reason to interfere with the normal process'[1]. However, assessment of risk must continue throughout pregnancy and labor: 'At any moment early complications may become apparent and induce the decision to refer the woman to a higher level of care . . .'[1]. By emphasizing the need for ongoing surveillance of maternal and fetal well-being, WHO answers many of the concerns resulting from the impossibility of predicting which low-risk women will remain low-risk throughout labor and birth.

Although midwives are considered to be specialists in normal childbearing, Gould has pointed out that midwives have never defined the constituents of normal labor[2]. She proposes a definition similar to that of WHO, but adds two other attributes: strenuous physical work by the mother; and movement by both the mother (seeking comfort and progress) and the fetus (through the birth canal). Gould believes 'movement and the notion of hard physical work to be crucial to a midwifery understanding of normal labor . . .' (page 424). Consequences of a normal labor, as defined by Gould, include psychosocial outcomes: a healthy mother and baby who are ready to adjust together to their new roles in continuing the lifecycle of the woman and the family; empowerment of the woman, and a sense of achievement that comes from her productive efforts and her active central (rather than passive) role in her child's birth. Gould believes that acceptance of this definition of normal birth would lead to improved care of women and a reversal of the prevailing cultural trend of increasing medicalization of birth.

Although neither WHO nor Gould emphasizes the rate of labor progress in their definitions of normal labor, numerous authors consider adequate labor progress to be a defining characteristic and a major focus of intrapartum care, along with monitoring and maintaining the well-being of mother and fetus. Given the wide range of normality, however, it is not surprising that 'there is no consensus as to what abnormal progress means[3],' and even less on how to prevent, identify, and correct this troublesome problem.

WHAT IS DYSFUNCTIONAL LABOR?

The term 'dysfunctional labor' is a catch-all term that refers to protracted or arrested progress in cervical dilation during the active phase of labor, or protracted or arrested descent during the second stage. Other terms, such as 'labor dystocia', 'uterine inertia', 'persistent malposition', 'cephalo-pelvic disproportion', 'failure to progress', 'protracted labor', and, as some clinicians have said in frustration, 'WCO' ('won't come out!'), have been used to refer to dysfunctional labor. In fact, Friedman compiled a list of 65 terms used to describe abnormal labor[4]! Some caregivers are less patient than others, and make the diagnosis of dysfunctional labor more quickly.

Diagnosis and management of dysfunctional labor vary, depending on the philosophy of the care provider[5]. For example, proponents of 'active management of labor' begin high dose oxytocin augmentation of nulliparas any time after labor is diagnosed, if the rate of dilation is less than 1 cm per hour for 2 hours[6]. Friedman's graphic analyses of labor progress, published between the mid-1950s and the 1970s, have profoundly influenced obstetrics in America and elsewhere for decades. He defined dysfunctional labor as the rate of dilation found in the lowest fifth percentile of his large study samples, which was less than 1.2 cm per hour in nulliparas, and less than 1.5 cm per hour in multiparas during the active phase of labor (from >3 cm to 10 cm)[4].

Zhang and others[7] suggest that Friedman's diagnostic criteria for dysfunctional labor are 'too stringent' to apply to today's childbearing women, who are larger in stature and have larger babies than the women of one or two generations ago, who were the subjects in Friedman's studies. Furthermore, when compared to Friedman's population, laboring women today receive oxytocin augmentation and epidural analgesia much more often. Zhang and colleagues propose that new criteria are needed, which allow a slower rate of dilation before resorting to cesarean delivery. They recently analyzed the partograms of almost 1200 nulliparas who had vaginal births, and compared their labor curves to Friedman's. They found substantial differences, especially between 4 and 6 cm, during which their median rate of dilation was actually the same as Friedman's 'dysfunctional' rate (1.2 cm per hour). Furthermore, the average duration of active labor (from 4 to 10 cm) was 5.5 hours, as opposed to Friedman's 2.5 hours[7].

Albers and colleagues conducted two studies of the length of labor in a total of 3984 healthy women at term, who did not receive oxytocin or epidural analgesia[8–9]. The women in both studies were cared for by nurse-midwives in either one hospital (in the first study) or in nine different hospitals (in the second study). Mean duration of active labor was similar in both studies: 7.7 hours in nulliparas, and 5.6 hours for multiparas. Active phase labors lasting as long as 19.4 hours in nulliparas and 13.8 hours in multiparas were associated with healthy outcomes. Albers and colleagues call for revision of clinical expectations for the length of active labor[8–9].

These findings support the approach used by those who diagnose dysfunctional labor only after the active phase has commenced and the rate of dilation is less than 0.5 cm per hour[5]. If the woman can be made comfortable and the fetus appears to be in no distress, they feel less urgency to speed progress. Unfortunately, non-clinical factors often dictate the caregiver's decision on when, whether, and how to intervene, for example the adequacy of staffing now and later, their own availability, their personal threshold for patience, and the woman's needs or desires.

Many midwives and others embrace a 'tolerance for wide variations in normal labor'[10]. They try to preserve normality and avoid the need for augmentation with oxytocin by ensuring the privacy of the woman, by remaining physically present but unobtrusive, by nourishing the woman, by supporting and reassuring her, by using non-pharmacological interventions (bath, movements, etc.), and by exercising patience and watchful waiting while allowing the labor process to unfold at its own pace.

MAINTAINING LABOR PROGRESS: PREVENTION OF DYSFUNCTIONAL LABOR

The first principle in management of labor dystocia is prevention. Many causes of dysfunctional labor exist (See Table 2.1). Some are detectable before labor begins, and some of these are correctable. For example, identifying fetal malposition (especially the occiput posterior, OP) in late pregnancy provides opportunities to rotate the fetus before labor. In fact, because fetal malposition is a major cause of labor dystocia[11], and labor dystocia is the leading indication for primary cesareans, it seems obvious that high priority should be placed on diagnosing the OP fetus and instituting measures to rotate the fetus during labor. Chapter 3 provides a variety of ways to identify the fetus' position, and measures intended to rotate the fetus before labor.

Table 2.1 Etiologies of dysfunctional labor (dystocia).

Etiology	Description	Comments
Cervical dystocia	Posterior unripe cervix at labor onset, scarred, fibrous cervix or 'rigid os'	Unripe cervix may prolong latent phase. Surgical scarring, damage from disease, or structural abnormality may increase cervical resistance
Emotional dystocia	Maternal distress or fear, exhaustion, severe pain	Increased catecholamine production may inhibit contractions
Fetal dystocia	Malposition, asynclitism, large or deflexed head, lack of engagement	Pendulous abdomen, size and shape of pelvis or fetal head may predispose fetus to malposition. Molding may enable vaginal birth
Iatrogenic dystocia	Misdiagnosis of labor or 2nd stage, inappropriate oxytocin use, maternal immobility, drugs, dehydration, disturbance	Misdiagnosis or unneeded interventions can slow or interfere with labor progress
Pelvic dystocia	Malformation, pelvic shape other than gynecoid, small dimensions	Maternal movement and upright positions increase pelvic dimensions
Uterine dystocia	Inadequate, or inefficient contractions	May be secondary to fear, fasting, dehydration, supine position, CPD, lactic acidosis in myometrium, or structural abnormalities

A role for the fetus in regulating labor?

Although scientific evidence is lacking, many maternity care professionals relate anecdotes of slow-progressing labors, which, when augmented with oxytocin, resulted in fetal distress and a cesarean. One wonders whether practitioners who tolerate slower progress in labor avoid cesareans for fetal distress that might be created if they augmented with oxytocin. The question of whether the fetus, perhaps through catecholamine production or some other means, influences the labor pattern is intriguing and may merit further scientific investigation.

THE PSYCHO-EMOTIONAL STATE OF THE WOMAN: REDUCING MATERNAL DISTRESS

By keeping in mind the psycho-emotional, physical, and physiological factors that are important in maintaining good labor progress, the caregiver can often prevent dystocia. Labor progress is facilitated when a woman feels safe, respected, and cared for by the experts who are responsible for her clinical safety, when she can remain active and upright, and when her pain is adequately and safely managed. Her partner or loved ones and her caregivers contribute significantly to such feelings. The opposite feelings of shame or embarrassment, of being observed, of feeling unsafe, being immobile, being treated with disrespect, feeling ignored or insignificant, may elicit a psychobiological reaction that interferes with efficient progress in labor.

Michel Odent, MD, an observer and student of normal birth since the early 1960s, has postulated that when women give birth 'in the method of the mammals' (that is, instinctively), their labors are more likely to proceed without difficulty. He postulates that when the neocortex, the newer and more uniquely human part of the brain (the thinking reasoning part) is overstimulated, the birth process is inhibited. Because the birth process involves coordinated activity within the endocrine system and the 'older', more primitive parts of the brain that humans share with other mammals, Odent advocates modifying present-day facilities and care practices to minimize stimulation of the neocortex. He notes that other mammals seek privacy in a comfortable, cozy, quiet space, and dim light when they are about to give birth. Such an environment for humans would reduce activity in the neocortex and allow the midbrain and brainstem to set in motion

Maternal Effects of Anxiety ('Tend and Befriend' Response) in Labor

Excessive maternal catecholamine levels in first stage of labor
Physiological response in mother: decreased blood flow to
uterus, decreased uterine contractions, increased duration
of first stage of labor, decreased blood flow to placenta
Physiological response in fetus: increased fetal production
of catecholamines, fetal conservation of oxygen, fetal heart
rate decelerations
Maternal psychological response: increased negative or
pessimistic perception of words and events by woman,
increased need for reassurance & support, protectiveness
towards fetus

2

Excessive catecholamine levels in second stage labor
Same fetal effects as listed above, 'Fetal ejection reflex'
(rapid expulsion of fetus)

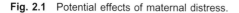

Fig. 2.1 Potential effects of maternal distress.

the processes, mediated by prostaglandins and hormones, that allow labor to proceed, undisturbed. Odent points out that in today's maternity facilities, the neocortex is constantly stimulated with bright lights, strangers, many questions, unfamiliar sights and sounds, etc., and optimal functioning of the primitive brain is inhibited, thus contributing to dystocia[12–13].

The well-known 'fight or flight' response, a physiological process that promotes survival of the endangered or frightened animal or human, is initiated by the outpouring of catecholamines or stress hormones, such as epinephrine (adrenalin), norepinephrine (noradrenalin), cortisol, and others. Triggered by physical danger, fear, anxiety, or other forms of distress, the fight or flight response has the potential of slowing labor progress (Fig. 2.1). During most of the first stage of labor, excessively high levels of circulating catecholamines cause maternal blood to be shunted away from the uterus, placenta, and other organs not essential for immediate survival, to the heart, lungs, brain, and skeletal muscle, the organs essential to

2

fight or flight. The decreased blood supply to the uterus and placenta slows uterine contractions[14] and decreases the availability of oxygen to the fetus[15]. Fear or anxiety also causes the woman to interpret caregivers' words or labor events in a pessimistic or negative way. Avoidance or reduction of maternal psychological distress or enhancement of the woman's sense of well-being appears to facilitate the physiological labor process. Interestingly, an outpouring of catecholamines in late first stage or close to birth has the opposite effect of speeding the birth by causing the 'fetal ejection reflex'[16]. In fact, many women briefly exhibit fear, anger, or even euphoria, typical catecholamine responses, just before the birth[12–13].

A recent review of studies of the fight or flight response reported differences between the behavioral responses of males and females when in physical danger or emotional distress[17]. While 'fight or flight may characterize the primary physiological responses to stress', the authors propose that, 'behaviorally, females' responses are more marked by a pattern of "tend-and-befriend"', which refers to protecting their young from harm, and reaching out for help, or affiliating with others to reduce the risks to themselves and their offspring.

Observations of laboring women and some research support these tend-and-befriend behaviors. Women want and need supportive people around them during labor. In fact, the absence of this kind of support is one of the most frequently mentioned reasons for later dissatisfaction with childbirth[18], and is commonly associated with post-traumatic stress disorder after childbirth[19–22]. A woman's protectiveness toward her child is evident; when she is told by a respected caregiver that her baby is in danger, she will quickly agree to whatever treatment is suggested, even if it does not fit with her prior expectations for her birth. On the other hand, if she does not trust the caregiver, she may try to protect her child by resisting suggested treatments.

Following are measures a caregiver may use to enhance the woman's feelings of security and trust, and reduce the likelihood of emotional distress.

Psycho-emotional measures

Before labor

Before birth, in childbirth classes, and in conversations with her midwife or doctor, encourage each woman to think about personally comforting things she and her partner might do or have available in labor, for example favorite music, scents, pictures, loved ones or a doula, her own clothing to wear during labor, visualizations, massage, or relaxation techniques. Such things may contribute to her personal comfort in the birth environment. Of course, most of these are easily available in a home birth, but will require some advanced planning and/or packing for a hospital birth.

Encourage parents to write a letter or 'birth plan' to the staff, introducing themselves and describing their concerns, fears, preferences, and choices regarding their care[23]. Ask to review and discuss the birth plan with the woman during a prenatal appointment. This provides an opportunity to communicate as equals, identify and clear up misunderstandings, and establish trust. If, as in the USA and Canada (and some parts of the UK), the nurse and midwife or doctor are strangers to the woman, they should check her chart for her psychosocial history, her birth plan, and clinical notes.

During labor: tips for nurses and midwives, especially when meeting the woman for the first time

- Introduce yourself by name, and call her by name. Greet her and her support team and orient them as appropriate to her needs and stage of labor. Introduce her to the unit (room, lighting, use of bed, bath or shower, call buttons, kitchen, nurses' station, lounge). Try to convey a sense of hospitality and friendliness, along with safety and competence.

- Ask about her plans and preferences. Try to be supportive of her wishes. Does she have a birth plan or preference list? If her wishes are somewhat unrealistic, discuss them kindly and respectfully, offering the choices you can provide[23]. Sometimes a detailed or negative birth plan reflects fear and mistrust of the staff. Try to reassure the woman and create rapport.

- Encourage an atmosphere of privacy, comfort, and intimacy between her and her support people:
  - knock before entering and keep door closed
  - do not leave her body exposed
  - tell her what comfort devices you have available (ice pack, hot pack, warm blankets, birth ball, beanbag chair, bath, shower, squatting bar, music, juices, tea, others)

- ○ encourage cuddling, hugging, 'slow dancing'
- ○ encourage and reassure the woman and remain with her as much as she wishes and as your other responsibilities allow

- Explain any clinical procedures or tests. Give her the results. If the woman's vital signs, her labor progress, and the fetal heart rate appear normal, it is reassuring to tell her so.

- Inform her of the signs of progress as you identify them. See pages 87–89 for information on the six ways to progress.

- Suggest comfort measures to help her cope with labor.

- Reassure her, not only with words, but also, as culturally appropriate, with praise, smiles, touch, hand-holding, or gestures of kindness and respect.

These measures create an atmosphere in which the woman feels well cared for and they have the added advantages of taking little time and costing next to nothing.

Physical comfort measures

Using simple physical comfort measures may increase the woman's sense of mastery and reduce her stress and the likelihood of a labor-slowing fight or flight response.

- Create an atmosphere (privacy, no sudden noises, dim light) that encourages the woman's spontaneous self-comforting behaviors and those learned in childbirth class:
  - ○ relaxation techniques/rhythmic movements
  - ○ calming vocalizations (moans, sighs)
  - ○ breathing techniques (see Chapter 8, pages 283–285)
  - ○ guided imagery/visualization

- Give her partner suggestions to use as long as they are acceptable to the woman:
  - ○ massage
  - ○ timing contractions or counting her breaths through each one to help her know where she is in the contraction (middle or end)
  - ○ encouraging rhythm in her movements, breathing, moaning, even mental activities

- ○ wiping her face and neck with a cool damp cloth
- ○ giving words of praise, encouragement
- ○ speaking in a soothing low rhythmic tone of voice
- Encourage the woman or couple to use available amenities, such as:
  - ○ hot or cold packs
  - ○ bath or shower
  - ○ birth ball
  - ○ cold or hot beverages, ice chips
  - ○ lounge
  - ○ tape or compact disc player, television

2

Physiological measures

The following basic physiological measures also tend to prevent underlying factors that can lead to dystocia.

- Encourage her to empty her bladder every hour or two. A distended bladder may increase pain or interfere with descent. Contractions sometimes reduce one's awareness of a full bladder, so she may need to be reminded.

- Make sure the woman remains well hydrated, but not over-hydrated. Oral liquids are a simple, comforting way to quench the woman's thirst. Have a variety of juices, frozen juice bars, teas, and water available for oral hydration. Numerous sources agree that there is no evidence of harm to healthy laboring women from drinking fluids during labor. Nor is there evidence that most women need intravenous (IV) fluids to prevent dehydration. Aspiration of gastric contents in the event of general anesthesia is not a valid reason to withhold liquids from healthy low-risk laboring women[5,24–27], even those with epidurals[28]. Nevertheless, it remains the policy or custom in many North American and British hospitals to restrict oral food and fluids, even in healthy uncomplicated pregnancies, and to give IV fluids instead[26–27]. Until those policies are changed, be sure that you do not cause overhydration with a too rapid intravenous infusion of fluids.

- Encourage the woman to seek comfort, that is, to try a variety of movements and positions and use ones that feel better to her. The most comfortable movements and positions seem to be ones that also enhance labor progress[29–30]. There is psychological benefit, and possible improvement in labor progress, without evidence of harm when healthy women move around during labor[30].

- Encourage the woman to relax her voluntary muscles, particularly those in her buttocks, pelvic floor, thighs, abdomen, and lower back.

WHY FOCUS ON MATERNAL POSITION?

In late pregnancy, changes in hormone production relax the ligaments and cartilage of the pelvic joints, allowing greater mobility in the sacroiliac joints and the pubic symphysis[31–33]. Pelvic mobility allows for subtle changes in the shape and size of the pelvis, which may facilitate an optimal position of the fetal head in the first stage, as well as the cardinal movements of flexion, internal rotation, and fetal descent in the second stage.

Changes in the woman's position may have beneficial effects on the following:

(1)   Alignment of pelvic bones and resulting shape and capacity of the pelvis[31–33].
(2)   Frequency, length, and efficiency of contractions[29–30].
(3)   'Drive angle' (Figs 2.2a, b), that is, the angle formed by the axis of the fetus' spine and the axis of the birth canal[34].
(4)   Effects of gravity[29–30].
(5)   Oxygen supply to fetus[29].

Frequent position changes in labor optimize the chance of a 'good fit' between the fetus and maternal pelvis (helping resolve occiput posterior position, asynclitism, and deflexion). Women often describe less pain when the fetus and pelvis are better aligned, an added benefit. Continuous movement (pelvic rocking, swaying, walking) results in continuing changes in the relationship of the pelvic bones to one another and the shape of the pelvis, which may serve to 'nudge' the fetus into a more favorable position.

No single position is optimal for all situations or for hours at a time. Therefore, the woman should be encouraged to move and try various positions and not to remain in one position for long periods when there is no apparent progress.

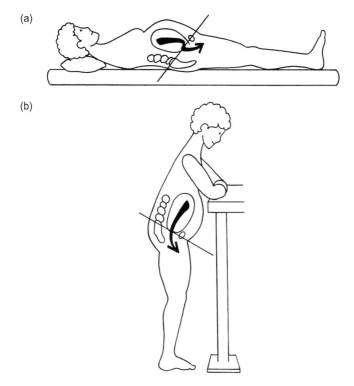

Fig. 2.2 Drive angle – (a) supine, (b) standing. (Adapted from reference 34).

This book contains descriptions of various maternal positions and movements that may help in specific situations. See the Toolkit in Chapter 7 for a detailed description and discussion of each position and movement.

MONITORING THE MOBILE WOMAN'S FETUS

There sometimes appears to be a trade-off between the advantages of maternal mobility and the presumed advantages of continuous electronic fetal monitoring (EFM), which usually requires the mother to remain lying in bed or semi-sitting. This trade-off can be resolved in a variety of ways. One way is to discontinue the routine practice of continuous EFM, because it carries virtually no benefit for the low-risk woman or baby, and some added risks[35]. For years it was assumed that continuous EFM improved newborn outcomes, but numerous scientific trials have failed to confirm that assumption; in fact, these trials found that there were disadvantages associated with EFM, such as an increase in cesareans and instrumental deliveries, with no improvement in newborn outcomes for women at low risk (and who are not receiving oxytocin)[5,35].

Auscultation

The findings of these trials led the professional organizations of obstetricians, in the USA (American College of Obstetricians and Gynecologists), Canada (Society of Obstetricians and Gynecologists), and the UK (Royal College of Obstetricians and Gynaecologists), during the late 1980s and early 1990s, to support or promote inter-mittent auscultation as either equal to, or preferred over electronic fetal monitoring, for low risk women with healthy pregnancies[36-38]. Each organization describes similar specific protocols for intermittent auscultation, and offers strict guidelines on circumstances that re-quire continuous electronic fetal monitoring and/or fetal scalp blood sampling.

When electronic fetal monitoring is required: options to enhance maternal mobility

Despite these endorsements of intermittent auscultation, EFM has become well established in most hospitals in the USA, UK, and Canada. A high percentage still monitor continuously, even when the women are at low risk. Many doctors, nurses, and midwives who were trained in reading electronic monitor tracings remain uneasy with auscultation. In many cases, the nurse or midwife may work in an institution where policies or doctors' orders require continuous EFM, and the women, despite the doctrines of informed consent and informed choice, have little say on this issue. There are also high-risk situations in which continuous EFM is called for. Is there anything that can be done to minimize the restriction to bed and the immobility that often accompany EFM?

The answer is yes.

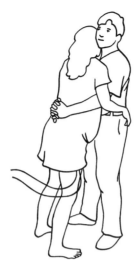

Fig. 2.3 Slow dancing with EFM.

Continuous EFM

The woman does not have to remain in any single position or in bed. She may lie on her side, sit up, kneel and lean forward, get out of bed and rock in a chair, stand and lean over the bed or a birth ball on the bed, sway or 'slow dance' (Fig. 2.3) with her partner beside the monitor, kneel, lunge, or even sit in the bath. (The Toolkit in Chapter 7 describes many of these techniques.)

Even if the fetal heart rate is easier to detect in one particular position, the woman should never be required to remain in that position for any longer than the time needed to document the heart rate. The woman's support person may be enlisted to hold the transducer in place (Fig. 2.4) or a washcloth may be placed between the transducer and its belt (Fig. 2.5) or mesh garment, so that it will not slip when the woman is in a standing, hands-and-knees, or other position. An internal scalp electrode usually has the advantage of not slipping out of place when the woman rolls over, kneels or squats (Fig. 2.6), as the external monitor may. However, the scalp electrode is more invasive than the external ultrasound transducer, requires ruptured membranes, and is more likely to promote maternal – fetal transmission

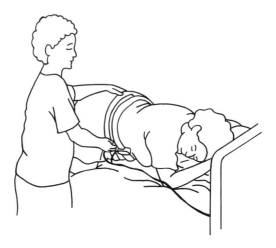

Fig. 2.4 Partner holding transducer in place.

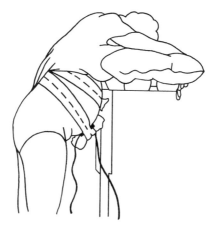

Fig. 2.5 Washcloth used to press transducer more firmly in place.

of Human Immunodeficiency Virus (HIV) in an HIV positive mother. Because ultrasound devices are being improved, there is now less reliance on internal electronic fetal monitoring. When an intrauterine pressure catheter (IUPC) is being used, a woman can

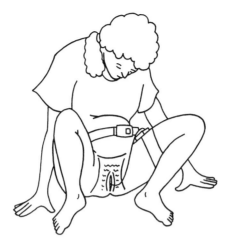

Fig. 2.6   Squatting with scalp electrode in place.

also make use of upright positions, but it may require adjustment of the pressure gauge when the woman changes positions, in order to maintain accurate pressure readings. One should ask how important it is to record intrauterine pressure, and avoid it if there are no compelling clinical reasons to do so.

Intermittent EFM

Some caregivers feel untrusting of their skills in auscultation, but do feel comfortable with intermittent EFM. The nurse or caregiver can merely hold the ultrasound transducer on the woman's belly for a minute or so every 15 minutes. The heart rate tracing will print out and may be easier to interpret for those who prefer a visible printout, along with the auditory transmission. For women who prefer to spend part of their labor in the bath, there are waterproof hand-held Doppler stethoscopes. Midwives who practice in out-of-hospital birth settings often use such devices. If not available in the hospital, the ultrasound transducer that comes with the electronic fetal monitor can also be used while the woman is immersed in water (Fig. 2.7). Check with your monitor manufacturer and your hospital's engineering department for assurance that there are no dangerous electronics in

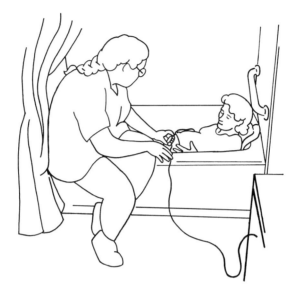

Fig. 2.7   Monitoring with a waterproof hand-held Doppler.

the transducer that can harm the woman or destroy the monitor when it is immersed in water (Chapter 8, p. 255).

Telemetry

If the woman must be monitored continuously and the birth setting has an EFM telemetry unit, the woman may walk in or outside her room or sit in the bath or shower (Figs 2.8, 2.9). The telemetry system consists of the same belts and transducers that come with standard EFM. These are connected to a portable radio transmitter that either clips to the woman's robe or hangs over the side of the bath. In a newer telemetry system both the ultrasound transducer and the contraction sensor contain small transmitters. These are held on the woman's trunk with elastic belts. All parts are watertight and safe to use in the bath or shower as shown in Figs 2.10 and 2.11. Again, check with the monitor manufacturer and your hospital engineering department to be sure that monitoring in the water is safe with your particular device.

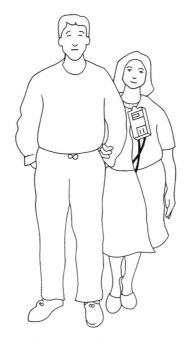

Fig. 2.8 Walking with telemetry monitor.

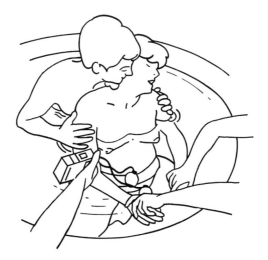

Fig. 2.9 Telemetry in bath.

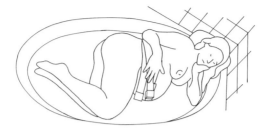

Fig. 2.10 Using wireless telemetry in bath.

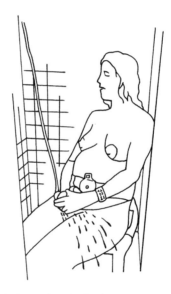

Fig. 2.11 Using wireless telemetry in shower.

Considering the documented benefits of walking and hydrotherapy in speeding slow progress and reducing pain[30], telemetry may be the optimal choice of monitoring methods when continuous monitoring is called for. (For more on the prevention of dystocia through movement and ambulation see pages 21–22 and Chapter 7, and for more on hydrotherapy see pages 252–257.)

By implementing these ideas, it may be possible to avoid some of the problems caused by immobility and the horizontal position that usually accompany electronic fetal monitoring. These problems may include persistent occiput posterior position, less efficient contractions, supine hypotension (if the woman remains on her back), and excessive pain.

TECHNIQUES TO ELICIT STRONGER CONTRACTIONS

2

The following techniques are associated with stronger or more frequent contractions.

- *Hydration*. Make sure that the woman is not dehydrated[22]. See page 21 for a discussion of hydration.
- *Movement and positioning*. If progress is slow, have the woman walk for half an hour, change positions frequently (about every half hour), and avoid the supine position.
- *Comforting touch*, such as stroking, backrubs, hand-holding, etc., may increase endogenous oxytocin production (Fig. 2.12).

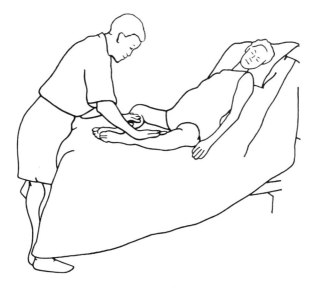

Fig. 2.12 Partner massaging woman's legs.

- *Nipple stimulation* done by either the woman or her partner can be used to stimulate contractions because it increases oxytocin production. The woman or her partner should start by stimulating one nipple, to see whether this will produce the desired effect. If not, both nipples may be stimulated. Contractions may become markedly longer and stronger so parents may need to be instructed to stop the nipple stimulation if contractions seem to become longer or stronger than is optimal for the fetus.
- *Acupressure* may be used to augment contractions. See Chapter 8, pages 259–260 for more information.
- *Warm compresses* or a hot water bottle placed on the fundus may augment contractions. See Chapter 8, page 275 for information on the use of heat.

CONCLUSION

In summary, this chapter describes practices that tend to prevent dystocia, with particular emphasis on minimizing maternal distress, promoting physiological measures that maintain progress, and encouraging movement and position changes by the woman.

REFERENCES

1. WHO (1996) Safe motherhood, Chapter 1. In: *Care in Normal Labor: A Practical Guide*. pp. 1–7. World Health Organization, Geneva.
2. Gould, D. (2000) Normal labour: a concept analysis. *Journal of Advanced Nursing* **31**, 418–27.
3. Cunningham, F., Gant, N., Leveno, K., Gilstrap III, L., Hauth, J. & Wenstrom, K. (editors) (2001) *Williams' Obstetrics*, 21st edn, p. 427. McGraw-Hill, New York.
4. Friedman, E. (1978) *Labor: Clinical Evaluation and Management*, 2nd edn. Appleton-Century-Crofts, New York.
5. Enkin, M., Keirse, M., Neilson, J., *et al.*, (2000) Monitoring the progress of labour. In: *A Guide to Effective Care in Pregnancy and Childbirth*, 3rd edn. Oxford University Press, Oxford.
6. O'Driscoll, K., Meagher, D. & Boylan, D. (1993) *Active Management of Labour*, 3rd edn. Mosby, London.
7. Zhang, J., Troendle, J., Yancey, M. (2002) Reassessing the labor curve in nulliparous women. *American Journal of Obstetrics and Gynecology*, **187**, 824–8.

8. Albers, L., Schiff, M. & Gorwoda, J. (1996) The length of active labor in normal pregnancies. *Obstetics and Gynecology*, **87**, 355–9.

9. Albers, L. (1999) The duration of labor in healthy women. *Journal of Perinatology*, **19**, 114–19.

10. Kennedy, H. & Shannon, M. (2004) Keeping birth normal: research findings on midwifery care during childbirth. *Journal of Obstetric, Gynecological and Neonatal Nursing*, **33**, 554–60.

11. Ponkey, S., Cohen, A., Heffher, L. & Lieberman, E. (2003) Persistent fetal occiput posterior position: obstetric outcomes. *Obstetrics and Gynecology*, **101** (5, Part 1), 915–920.

12. Odent, M. (1992) *The Nature of Birth and Breastfeeding*. Bergin & Garvey, Westport, Conn.

13. Odent, M. (1999) Birth reborn, Chapter 6. In: *The Scientification of Love*. Free Association Books, London.

14. Lederman, R.P., Lederman, E., Work, B.A. & McCann, D.S. (1981) Relationship of psychological factors in pregnancy to progress in labor. *Nursing Research*, **25**, 94–8.

15. Lederman, E., Lederman, R.P., Work, B.A. & McCann, D.S. (1981) Maternal psychological and physiologic correlates of fetal-newborn health status. *American Journal of Obstetrics and Gynecology*, **139**, 956–60.

16. Newton, N. (1987) The fetus ejection reflex revisited. *Birth*, **14** (2), 106–108.

17. Taylor, S., Klein, L., Lewis, B., Gruenewald, T., Gurung, R. & Updegraff, J. (2000) Biobehavioral responses to stress in females: Tend-and-befriend, not fight-or-flight. *Psychological Reviews*, **107**, 411–29.

18. Hodnett, E. (2002) Pain and women's satisfaction with the experience of childbirth: a systematic review. *American Journal of Obstettrics and Gynecology*, **186**, s160–172.

19. Creedy, D., Shochet, I. & Horsfall, J. (2000) Childbirth and the development of acute trauma symptoms: incidence and contributing factors. *Birth*, **27**, 104–111.

20. Soet, J., Brack, G. & Dilorio, C. (2003) Prevalence and predictors of women's experience of psychological trauma during childbirth. *Birth*, **30**, 36–46.

21. Czarnocka, J. & Slade, P. (2000) Prevalence and predictors of post-traumatic stress symptoms following childbirth. *British Journal of Clinical Psychology*, **39**, 35–51.

22. Beck, C. (2004) Post-traumatic stress disorder due to childbirth: the aftermath. *Nursing Research*, **53**, 216–224.

23. Simkin, P., Whalley, J. & Keppler, A. (2001) Planning for birth and postpartum, Chapter 7. In: *Pregnancy, Childbirth and the Newborn: The Complete Guide*. Meadowbrook Press, Minnetonka, Minnesota.

24. Sharp, D.A. (1997) Restriction of oral intake for women in labour. *British Journal of Midwifery*, **5** (7), 408–412.

25. The CNM Data Group. (1999) Clinical Bulletin: Intrapartum Nutrition. *Journal of Nursing and Midwifery*, **44** (3), 129–34.

26. Berry, H. (1997) Feast or famine? Oral intake during labour: current evidence and practice. *British Journal of Midwifery*, **5** (7), 413–17.

27. Sleutel, M. & Golden, S. (1999) Fasting in labor: relic or requirement. *Journal of Obstetrics, Gynecology and Neonatal Nursing*, **28**, 507–512.

28. American College of Obstetricians and Gynecologists (ACOG) (2002) ACOG Practice Bulletin: Obstetric Analgesia and Anesthesia. *Obstetrics and Gynecology*, **100**, 177–91.

29. Roberts, J. (1989) Maternal position during the first stage of labour. In: *Effective Care in Pregnancy and Childbirth*, vol. 2 (eds I. Chalmers, M. Enkin, & M.J.N.C. Keirse.) Oxford University Press, Oxford.

30. Simkin, P. & O'Hara, M. (2002) Nonpharmacologic relief of pain during labor: systematic reviews of five methods. *American Journal of Obstetrics and Gynecology*, **186**, s131–59.

31. Russell, J.G.B. (1969) Moulding of the pelvic outlet. *Journal of Obstetrics and Gynaecology, British Commonwealth*, **76**, 817–20.

32. Michel, S., Rake, A., Treiber, K., *et al.* (2002) MR obstetric pelvimetry: effect of birthing position on pelvic bony dimensions. *American Journal of Roentgenology*, **179**, 1063–7.

33. Simkin, P. (2003) Maternal positions and pelves revisited. *Birth*, **30**, 130–32.

34. Fenwick, L. & Simkin, P. (1987) Maternal positioning to treat dystocia. *Clinical Obstetrics and Gynecology*, **30**, 83–9.

35. Thacker, S., Stroup, D. & Chang, M. (2001) Continuous electronic heart rate monitoring for fetal assessment during labor (Cochrane Review). In: *The Cochrane Library*, Issue 3, 2004. Chichester, UK. John Wiley & Sons, Ltd.

36. AAP, ACOG (1988) *Guidelines for Perinatal Care*, 2nd edn. American Academy of Pediatrics and American College of Obstetricians and Gynecologists, Washington, DC.

37. Liston, R., Crane, J. & the SOGC Fetal Health Surveillance Working Group (2002) *Fetal Health Surveillance in Labour. Clinical Practice Guidelines*, **112**, 1–13. Society of Obstetricians and Gynecologists, Ottawa.

38. Royal College of Obstetricians and Gynaecologists (2001) *The Use of Electronic Fetal Monitoring. The Use and Interpretation of Cardiotocography in Intrapartum Fetal Surveillance*. (Evidence-based clinical guidelines, no. 8). Royal College of Obstetricians and Gynaecologists Press, London.

Chapter 3

Assessing Progress in Labor

by Suzy Myers, LM, CPM, MPH

Before labor begins, 36
Malposition, 36
Observing for clues to fetal position, 38
Palpating for fetal position, 39
Palpating using Leopold's maneuvers, 40
Auscultating for fetal position, 43
Belly mapping, 44
Other assessments prior to labor, 48
Assessments during labor, 50
Position, attitude and descent of the fetus, 50
Vaginal examinations: indications and timing, 51
Performing a vaginal examination during labor, 51
The vaginal exam, step by step, 53
Assessing the cervix, 54
Unusual cervical findings, 55
The presenting part, 56
The vagina and bony pelvis, 64
Quality of contractions, 64
Assessing the mother's condition, 67
Assessing the fetus, 69
How to perform intermittent auscultation, 70
Reassuring signs of fetal well-being that can be assessed without EFM, 72
Putting it all together, 75
Assessing progress in first stage, 75
Features of normal latent phase, 76
Features of normal active phase, 76
Assessing progress in second stage, 77
Features of normal second stage, 77
Conclusion, 77
References, 77

Many assessments exist to help determine when labor is progressing normally and when it is not. These assessments inform and guide midwives, physicians, and nurses in promoting normal labor progress, preventing dysfunctional labors, and treating dystocia appropriately when it occurs. While training, mentorship, and practice are required to master these assessment skills, this chapter will provide descriptions, rationale, and practical tips.

Readers of this book who have neither professional training in maternity nursing, midwifery or medicine, nor clinical responsibility for the health of pregnant or laboring women (i.e. doulas and childbirth educators) do not use the hands-on assessment techniques because they are outside their scope of practice. Doulas and childbirth educators may, however, find this chapter helpful in understanding the reasons for and meanings of these assessments.

This chapter addresses labor progress assessment with a full-term, singleton fetus in a longitudinal lie and a cephalic presentation (aligned vertically in the mother's torso, with the head lying over the pelvic inlet).

BEFORE LABOR BEGINS

Assessing fetal position before labor begins helps predict which labors may be more or less dysfunctional, and, more importantly, may provide an opportunity to correct some problems before labor begins.

Malposition

A primary cause of dysfunctional labor is fetal malposition[1]. During labor, fetal position is determined largely by palpating bony landmarks on the fetal head through a reasonably dilated cervix. In the last weeks of pregnancy, the location and orientation of the fetal back (towards the woman's front or back) can offer a presumptive, if not a positive, diagnosis of the occiput anterior or occiput posterior fetal position. Identifying the fetus who is in an occiput posterior position prior to labor may help prevent a painful or dystotic 'back' labor. By using exercises and positioning, the mother may be able to encourage the fetus to 'roll over' so that it is more likely to enter the pelvis in an occiput anterior position when labor begins[2-5].

Tools used to assess fetal position before labor include observation, palpation, and auscultation.

Table 3.1 Fetal positions – abdominal views. Fetal position is described by the location of the occiput (the back of the fetal head) in relation to the *mother's* left or right, and to the front (anterior) or back (posterior) of her pelvis, as shown in Table 3.1

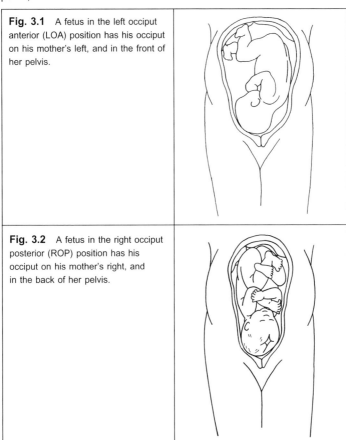

Fig. 3.1 A fetus in the left occiput anterior (LOA) position has his occiput on his mother's left, and in the front of her pelvis.

3

Fig. 3.2 A fetus in the right occiput posterior (ROP) position has his occiput on his mother's right, and in the back of her pelvis.

Table 3.1   (continued)

Fig. 3.3   A fetus in the left occiput transverse (LOT) position has his occiput on the mother's left side and in the middle between her front and back.

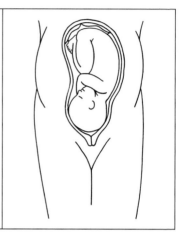

Observing for clues to fetal position

Observe the contour of the maternal abdomen with the woman lying on her back (to the extent that this is comfortable for her):

- When the fetus is lying with its back anterior (toward the woman's front), the maternal abdominal wall looks convex and the umbilicus may appear 'popped out' as in Fig. 3.4. The mother reports fetal movement predominantly in the upper quadrant opposite the fetal back.

- When the fetal back is oriented more posteriorly (toward the mother's spine), the abdomen looks concave, especially depressed in the region of the umbilicus or below, as shown in Fig. 3.5. The mother may report that she feels fetal movement in the mid-line, or 'everywhere'. These are signs that the fetus is more likely to enter the maternal pelvis in the less favorable occiput posterior position as shown in Fig. 3.2 in Table 3.1.

These observations may be difficult in women with large amounts of adipose tissue on their abdomens.

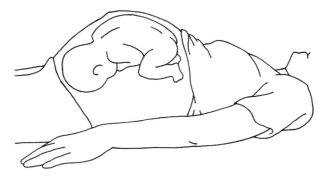

Fig. 3.4 Abdominal contour with fetal back anterior.

3

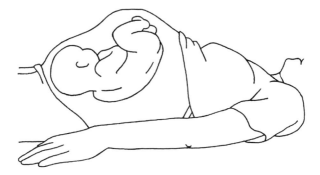

Fig. 3.5 Abdominal contour with fetal back posterior.

Palpating for fetal position

Careful palpation can help identify the orientation of the fetal back and those fetuses more likely to enter the pelvis in an occiput posterior position. (This is not relevant prior to 32–34 weeks, when the fetus is still relatively mobile.)

• When the fetal back is anterior, the side of the maternal abdomen where the back is located (left or right) feels smooth and firm, while on the opposite side fetal limbs ('small parts') are easily felt.

- When the fetal back is posterior, it may be difficult to palpate any smooth back. Fetal limbs may be palpated on either side of the midline.

Palpating using Leopold's maneuvers

Leopold's maneuvers are a systematic, four-step method for palpating the uterus to determine fetal lie, presentation, position, and engagement in the pelvis. Other information, such as uterine tone and estimated fetal weight, is also obtained by careful abdominal palpation in late pregnancy or during labor[6].

The technique

The woman should empty her bladder and then recline on a comfortable, firm surface, with her abdomen exposed. She should be helped to relax her abdominal muscles by bending her knees slightly, or resting them on a pillow. The clinical caregiver (midwife, nurse or doctor) should warm her or his hands, explain the procedure, and ask the mother to provide feedback if anything causes her discomfort. Generally, the clinical caregiver stands or kneels beside the examination surface: right-handed people on the woman's right, left-handed people on her left.

The four steps

The order of the following maneuvers is not important.

(1)   The first maneuver (Fig. 3.6) helps identify what part of the fetus is in the fundus (the top of the uterus). Facing the woman's head, the caregiver places both hands palm down on the woman's upper abdomen and, using firm but gentle pressure, feels the fundus and the height, shape, size, and consistency of the fetal parts in that area. When the lie is longitudinal and the presentation is cephalic, the breech is palpated in the fundus. It may feel bony and relatively large, but is differentiated from the head by feeling continuous with the spine and moving with it. In contrast, when the head is in the fundus (breech presentation), it usually feels ballotable, that is, it 'bounces' between the palpating hands because it is on the neck,

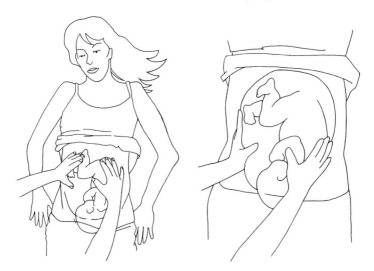

Fig. 3.6 Leopold's Maneuver # 1.   **Fig. 3.7** Leopold's Maneuver # 2.

and can be moved independently from the fetal back. When the lie is transverse, neither a head nor a breech can be palpated in the fundus.

(2) The second maneuver (Fig. 3.7) helps determine the location of the fetal back. Still facing the woman's head, the caregiver places her or his hands, palm down, on either side of the woman's abdomen. By keeping both hands in contact with the abdomen, and alternating pressure from one hand to the other, the caregiver can palpate the shape and bulk of fetal parts on either side of the maternal torso and around toward the maternal spine. With this maneuver, the caregiver may differentiate the feel of smooth back from knobby limbs ('small parts'), and amniotic fluid from fetal body parts. When the lie is transverse, the head or breech may be palpated on one or the other side of the maternal torso.

The final two Leopold's maneuvers are used to confirm the presentation and lie and to assess the presenting part and its descent into the pelvis.

(3) For the third maneuver (Fig. 3.8), the caregiver uses the thumb and forefinger of the dominant hand to gently palpate

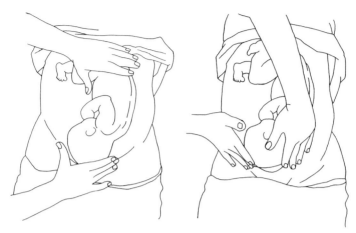

Fig. 3.8   Leopold's Maneuver # 3.   **Fig. 3.9**   Leopold's Maneuver # 4.

the lower pole of the uterus, just above the symphysis. The non-dominant hand may be used to grasp the fundus at the same time. If the lie is longitudinal and the presenting part is cephalic, the examiner should feel the large bony skull, which is often mobile if not yet deeply engaged. If the presenting part is the breech, although it may feel bony, it is much smaller than the head and does not move independently of the body. When the lie is transverse, the lower pole, like the fundus, feels empty of fetal parts.

(4)   For the fourth maneuver (Fig. 3.9) the examiner turns to face the woman's feet, and places one hand on each side of the woman's abdomen. With the fingers pointing toward the woman's feet, the caregiver presses the fingertips gently and firmly towards the maternal spine and around the presenting part. A term head that is floating above the pelvic brim is easily palpated. It feels round, large and mobile. As the head descends into the bowl of the pelvic inlet it becomes more difficult to palpate. When the fetal head is deeply engaged prior to labor, it may be nearly impossible to feel on external palpation, and sometimes requires internal assessment or an ultrasound to confirm a cephalic presentation.

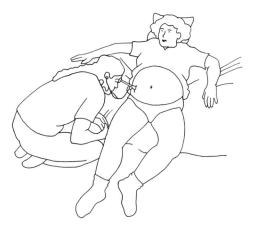

Fig. 3.10 Auscultating fetal heart tones with a fetoscope.

Auscultating for fetal position

In most fetuses near term, the loudest sounds of the fetal heart are heard through the fetal back, at approximately the level of the scapula or shoulders. Locating this point of maximum intensity of the fetal heart tones helps determine the orientation of the fetal back, either anterior or posterior. The best tool for this purpose is a fetoscope (such as the Leff or De Lee-Hillis fetoscope, or the Pinard horn), which allows for direct auscultation of the fetal heart, (Fig. 3.10) rather than a Doppler. (Dopplers use ultrasound to create an artificial sound that is not affected by proximity to the heart valves.)

When a cephalic fetus near term is oriented with his back curved towards the mother's front, the heart tones are crisp and clear, and are easily heard on the side of the maternal abdomen where the fetal back lies, below the maternal umbilicus and several centimeters from the midline, (LOA or ROA in Fig. 3.11). When the fetus is oriented with his back curved towards the mother's spine, the point of maximum intensity is in the right or left lateral area of the maternal abdomen (LOP or ROP in Fig. 3.11). Rarely, if the fetal back is in a concave position with the head completely extended (face presentation), the fetal heart tones may be heard through the fetal chest, sounding muffled, distant and difficult to hear[6].

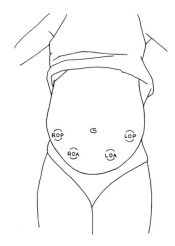

Fig. 3.11 Location of fetal heart tones with fetus in ROP, ROA, LOA, and LOP.

Belly Mapping

Belly mapping is a three-step process conceived by Gail Tully to identify fetal position, integrating mothers' observations, palpation, and auscultation of the fetal heart. It is an effective way to record the fetal position and explain it to mothers. Midwives, doctors and nurses find it helpful to combine belly mapping with Leopold's maneuvers to involve women in their care and enhance communications. We include here a description of this process, condensed from her 2005 book, *Spinning Babies: Childbirth Made Easier with Fetal Positioning* (Maternity House Publishing, Bloomington, Minn., USA).

Step 1: make a pie
Belly Mapping involves mentally dividing the maternal abdomen into quadrants ('pie pieces'), and drawing it on paper as shown in Fig. 3.B1.

The woman can often contribute much of the information needed to identify the position of her fetus, including:

- Which side of her belly is firm (if either)
- Where she feels the 'big bulge' of the fetal buttocks or head
- Where she feels stronger kicks (fetal feet or knees)
- Where she feels stretching from fetal leg movements
- Where she feels smaller movements (hands, elbows)

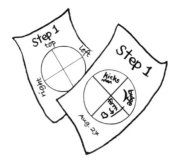

Fig. 3.B1 'Pie' map form.

Fig. 3.B2 shows a woman's experiences and how the belly map represents them.

The midwife, doctor or nurse uses clinical skills (Leopold's maneuvers, auscultation, and possibly ultrasound) to confirm and/or add to the mother's subjective information on fetal position, and marks all this in more detail on the belly map. (The 'heart' represents where fetal heart tones are heard using a fetoscope or Pinard horn. Because Doppler ultrasound fetoscopes can detect fetal heart tones farther from their point of origin, they are not as useful for this purpose.)

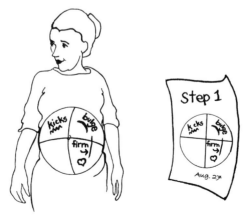

Fig. 3.B2 Example of a belly map.

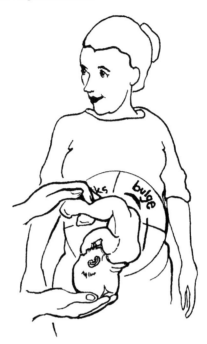

Fig. 3.B3   Using a doll to explain the position.

Step 2: visualize the baby
Putting all the information together, the care provider gets a good picture of the baby in the womb. When they are certain of the fetal position, some providers actually draw an outline of the fetus on the woman's abdomen with a non-toxic marker so that she can visualize how her baby is positioned. Or they may position a fetal doll over her abdomen to show the woman how her baby is positioned (Fig. 3.B3).

Step 3: name the position
Both the woman and her care provider will gain a clear picture of the fetus' position and will be able to discuss it. Figs 3.B4 and 3.B5 show the correlation between belly maps, see-through views, and fetus-in-the-pelvis views for fetuses in left occiput anterior (LOA) and right occiput posterior (ROP).

   If the provider identifies an unfavorable position in late pregnancy, the mother may be able to use maternal positioning and exercises to

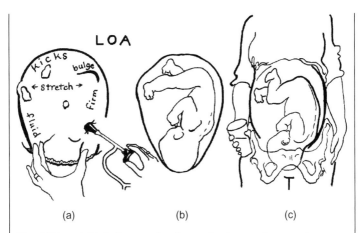

Fig. 3.B4   a LOA belly map showing mother's experience and clinician's findings, b LOA fetus, c LOA fetus in the pelvis.

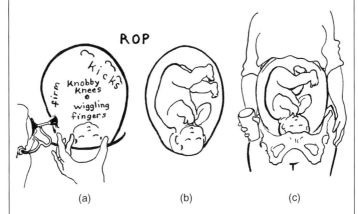

Fig. 3.B5   a ROP belly map showing mother's experience and clinician's findings, b ROP fetus, c ROP fetus in the pelvis.

reposition the fetus before labor. These may be more successful if they can be done in the last weeks of pregnancy before the fetal head is engaged. Sutton[3] and Scott[4] have devised an approach, 'Optimal Fetal Positioning, (OFP)' that combines late pregnancy and intrapartum positions to facilitate and maintain favorable fetal positions. This popular approach should be studied scientifically for its effectiveness. Tully's *Spinning Babies* approach utilizes optimal fetal positioning concepts (pages 85–87) plus other positions, movements, and devices learned from traditional midwives, physical therapists, chiropractors, and her own original discoveries while working with laboring women. See Chapter 4 for more information on repositioning the fetus.

Illustrations in this text box copyright Gail N.Tully 2005, reprinted by permission from Tully, G.N. (2005) *Spinning Babies: Childbirth Made Easier with Fetal Positioning*, Maternity House Publishing, Bloomington Minn. USA.

3

Other assessments prior to labor

Estimating fetal weight

Although most women with large babies deliver them without difficulty[7], fetal macrosomia can complicate labor[1 and 8]. Additionally, when the fetus is large, problems associated with malposition may be compounded.

Methods of estimating fetal weight at term are imprecise. Fundal height measurement is a poor predictor of fetal weight, although it may be useful to screen for further investigation[9]. Ultrasound assessments and palpation have equivalent accuracy, with an estimated margin of error of +/- 10–20%. The accuracy of palpation is significantly increased when the examiner is experienced[10–11], but reduced when the fetus is macrosomic[8]. Furthermore, an inaccurate prediction of fetal macrosomia may influence a diagnosis of labor dysfunction, leading to cesarean delivery.[12]

The best way to refine palpation skills for estimating fetal weight is to practice Leopold's maneuvers on every available woman at term or in labor, commit oneself to an estimated fetal weight, and verify it when the baby is born.

The birth weight prediction equation

There may be promise in a 'birth weight prediction equation' described by Nahum[13]. Based on six maternal and pregnancy-specific characteristics, it predicted the birth weights of term, healthy Caucasian infants within an average of plus or minus 8%, better than ultrasound. For predicting macrosomia, the equation was equivalent to ultrasound.

To summarize, the value of estimating fetal weight is questionable because of these problems: current methods of predicting birth weight are not reliable; the impact of macrosomia is variable; and it is not possible to reverse excessive fetal weight at or near term. Nonetheless, when labor progress is poor, caregivers may use an estimation of fetal weight as just that: an *estimation*, and one of many variables factored in to the complex problem solving needed to help resolve dysfunctional labors.

Assessing the cervix prior to labor

During pregnancy, the cervix is composed of dense collagen fibers providing a firm, inelastic tubular structure that helps keep the uterine contents safely contained. In labor, the role of the cervix is reversed. It must become elastic enough for the muscular activity of the uterus to open it and expel the fetus. To accomplish this, the woman's body alters the composition of the cervical tissue. Collagen fibers break down, elastin fibers in the internal os provide stretch, and the water content of the connective tissue increases, making the cervix soft and stretchy. These changes, called cervical ripening, begin weeks before labor's onset, and are caused by hormonal influences distinct from the mechanisms of effacement and dilation.[14] Some labor problems, both preterm labors and prolonged labors at term, may be the result of *cervical* dysfunction, rather than *uterine* dysfunction, when the cervix undergoes these changes too soon or does not complete them[15-17].

In 1964 Bishop[18] published his 15-point scoring system for evaluating the 'induce-ability' of labor, based on five factors: cervical dilation, effacement, consistency, position in the vagina, and station of the head. A ripe, or favorable-for-induction cervix, has a Bishop's score of 6-8. The Bishop score has also been used more recently to assess the need for pre-induction cervical ripening agents.

It has become common for caregivers to use Bishop's five variables to evaluate the cervical ripeness of women who are not necessarily candidates for induction, sometimes with weekly routine cervical exams in the last month of pregnancy. How useful are these examinations? Assessing the pre-labor cervix in women at term may help identify those more likely to experience short or prolonged latent phases[19]. Many people agree that, especially in nulliparas, women who begin labor with cervices that are long, firm, closed, and posterior are more likely to experience prolonged latent phases, while those whose cervices are thin, stretchy, and partially dilated are likely to progress more rapidly to the active phase. However, the value of pre-labor cervical assessment in predicting the onset of labor or active phase disorders is not substantiated in any research literature.

It may be tempting to tell a woman whose cervix is soft, thin, anterior, and 2 cm dilated that she will surely be in labor the next day, or to tell a woman with a closed, uneffaced cervix that she will still be pregnant next week. However, the condition of the cervix late in pregnancy does not predict when labor will begin or how it will progress, and these statements are inaccurate often enough to cause patients unnecessary distress. The decision to examine the cervix before the onset of labor should be based on a balanced assessment of the value of the information provided and client preference, rather than routine.

The role of cervical ripening and compliance in the etiology of problem labor (both prolonged and preterm) deserves further study.

ASSESSMENTS DURING LABOR

It is important to assess labor progress holistically, taking into account the many complex factors and their interactions, which influence labor progress. These include:

- Position, attitude (whether the fetal chin is well flexed toward the chest) and descent of the fetus
- Cervical change over time
- Quality of contractions
- Condition of the mother
- Condition of the fetus

Position, attitude and descent of the fetus

These are assessed during labor using some of the tools described for prenatal assessment. In addition, more precise information is obtained via internal vaginal examinations. Vaginal examinations also provide essential information about cervical change when repeated over time.

Vaginal examinations: indications and timing

Each woman in labor should be treated individually and her labor assessed as her needs dictate. This means that, rather than being done in all labors at a predetermined time interval or according to a protocol, vaginal exams are done as the need arises, and with the woman's understanding and consent. Appreciating that this examination is a significant intrusion for most women, the caregiver should take time to establish rapport before performing a vaginal exam. Reasons that justify assessing labor progress using vaginal examinations include:

- At the beginning of caring for a woman, to establish a baseline so that future progress or lack of progress can be better assessed.
- When a period of time in active labor has elapsed, usually more than three hours, and the labor pattern does not seem to be progressing (contractions are not becoming longer, more frequent, or more intense) or when there are no other outward signs of progress (mother's affect, spontaneous bearing down efforts, etc.).
- After an intervention has been implemented for some time, to assess whether the desired effect has been achieved (e.g., a period of stair climbing to aid in rotation of the fetal head, or time in the bath).
- When the woman in labor requests an assessment of her progress, or expresses discouragement, or a desire for pain medication.
- When there is a spontaneous urge to push, without other signs of fetal descent over a reasonable time.
- When there are non-reassuring fetal heart rate changes or any other concerning signs, such as excess vaginal bleeding.
- When an internal monitor (scalp lead or intrauterine pressure catheter) is needed.

Performing a vaginal examination during labor

Preparing to do the examination

Ideally, caregivers are not only making clinical assessments, but are also mindful of the laboring woman's needs for emotional support and accurate information. The vaginal examination in labor should be approached with these principles in mind.

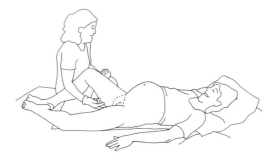

Fig. 3.12   Maternal position for vaginal examination.

First, it is helpful to sit with the woman and observe her labor pattern and her responses to it.

- What are the frequency, duration and quality of the contractions?
- How is the woman coping with them? (See Chapter 8, pages 265–266)
- Is she moving with, or between contractions?
- What positions does she spontaneously assume?

After making these basic observations, the caregiver should ask the woman if she thinks it would be helpful to assess her progress with a vaginal examination. Some women will welcome this information, while others are not yet ready. It is important to explain the benefits of having this information and not to act without her permission.

Ask the woman to empty her bladder before the exam. Next, she should lie down on a firm comfortable surface, preferably on her back with her head supported by not more than one pillow, as shown in Fig. 3.12. If lying on her back is too uncomfortable, she can rest in a supported semi-prone position with a pillow wedged under one hip. The mother's legs should be well supported, with her knees bent and wide apart, and the soles of her feet either together or flat on the bed's surface.

Some experienced practitioners perform vaginal exams with the mother in other positions (on hands and knees, standing, sitting, or squatting). This allows them to assess the station and cervical dilation. However, it is difficult to gain more detailed information, such as position of the presenting part, with the mother in these positions. When detailed information is needed it is better to ask the mother to lie down briefly than to have to repeat the exam.

After gaining the woman's permission, it is important to explain each step, offer to stop at any point if the woman requests it, and request her feedback about anything that hurts. The woman's ability to relax during this examination is important if the provider is to obtain the necessary information. But it is also a quality of care issue. Good care is defined as being both sensitive to the woman's needs and effective in obtaining the needed data. Some women experience fear during vaginal exams and may not be able to tolerate them, especially when performed by unfamiliar people or done without consideration of their discomfort. Often, these are women who have experienced previous trauma (i.e. sexual abuse or rough and inconsiderate vaginal exams). In order to be examined, they need patience, gentleness, and understanding from their providers, and a sense of being in control over whether, when, by whom, and how the exam will be done[20].

The vaginal exam, step by step

- The clinical caregiver washes and warms her or his hands, and starts with firm, but gentle abdominal palpation, using the basic Leopold's maneuvers.
  - As in the prenatal examination (pages 40–42), the caregiver determines the location and orientation of the fetal back (toward the woman's abdominal wall or toward her spine).
  - The caregiver estimates fetal weight, using palpation as well as historical information about the woman and her pregnancy. (Labor is the perfect opportunity to refine this skill – verifying the estimate will be possible very soon.)
  - The next step is to assess uterine tone, between and during contractions, by gently palpating at the fundus with the fingertips. (See Quality of contractions, pages 64–67).
  - This is also a good time to assess fetal heart rate and maternal vital signs. Consolidating necessary assessments allows the woman to labor undisturbed for longer periods.

- Next, the caregiver asks the woman's permission to begin the vaginal exam.

- Between contractions, the caregiver inserts first one (the fore-finger) and then two fingers (adding the middle finger) into the vagina, putting firm but gentle pressure on the posterior vaginal wall, and avoiding pressure on the urethra. At the same time, the examiner asks the mother to relax her vaginal muscles. Without the mother's cooperation and active relaxation, this exam may be uncomfortable for her, and accurate assessment may be difficult.

- If the fingers were inserted with the pads down, when they have reached the bulbo-cavernosus muscle, or about 3–4 cm into the vagina, the examiner explains that she or he will rotate the fingers so that the wrist is face up. This position allows for better assessment of the cervix, the presenting part, the vagina, and the pelvis.

3

Assessing the cervix

- Position: is the os anterior, posterior, or midline? When the cervical os is posterior, sometimes it is just possible to reach it, but not enough to assess dilation. In this case, the caregiver may be able, by applying gentle, steady pressure, to reach the os and manually pull it forward. Another aid is to ask the woman to place a fist under each buttock to help tilt the pelvis. This should bring the cervix into a more 'reachable' position.

- Consistency: are the cervical tissue and os stretchy and soft, or firm? As labor progresses, the cervix should become softer and more yielding. A thick, rigid cervix is abnormal.

- Effacement: how long is the cervical canal? It is difficult, if not impossible, to assess effacement digitally without being able to insert at least one finger into the cervix. Since the length of the cervix prior to labor varies from 1 to 4 cm, effacement is best expressed in terms of the length of the cervical canal, in centimeters or fractions of centimeters (rather than using the older method of expressing effacement as a percentage).[21] A completely effaced cervix is 'paper thin'.

- Dilation: how open is the cervix, measured in centimeters, without manual stretching? The first 6–7 cm are assessed by evaluating how open the cervix is. It takes practice to know the approximate number of finger breadths, or the distance between fingers, and the corresponding dilation. Practice tools include plastic models made for this purpose, as well as household objects, such as jars with various sized mouths. The last 3 cm (from 7 cm to fully dilated) are easier to assess, because they are measured by evaluating how much of the cervix remains on *one* side, between the open edge of the os and where the cervix meets the lower uterine segment. Although '10 cm' has been used to express complete dilation, measurable full dilation could vary between 9 and 12 cm depending on the diameters of the head.

- Membranes: are they intact or ruptured? A large bulging forebag is easy to feel and may make assessment of fetal position difficult. When there is no bulging bag of fluid presenting, the examiner should learn to discern the feel of the slippery membrane over the head as compared to the way the scalp feels when membranes are ruptured.

Unusual cervical findings

- The 'zipper' cervix: while the cervix is quite thin, the os is adherent and closed. Sometimes, after near complete effacement is achieved, this can be overcome by inserting one or two fingers and stretching the os open during a contraction. As the adhesion releases, the os opens like a zipper, sometimes dilating from 1 to 3 or 4 cm in one contraction. Expect bloody show as capillaries rupture with stretching.

- The rigid os: the cervix may be partially dilated, but has thickness and lacks a feeling of elasticity. It does not yield easily with contractions. This may be a sign of primary cervical dysfunction[15] or a consequence of edema in the cervix, caused by a poorly fitting head or uneven pressure on the cervix during contractions. In the former, the cervix never softens and effaces; in the latter, the cervix may be thinned and dilated during the latent phase or early active phase, but becomes swollen in late active phase.

- The os is not palpable at all. The lower uterine segment is thinned, the head is well applied with a low station, and exam findings may mimic full dilation. Sometimes, with careful examination, it is possible to find a small depression where the os is, but this author has encountered one case in which several experienced examiners were unable to locate even this landmark.

○ Persistent anterior cervical 'lip': This occurs when most of the cervix has retracted behind the head (no rim of cervix is palpated around the lateral or posterior aspects of the head), but the anterior portion of the cervix is caught between the head and the symphysis pubis. Position changes, time and patience usually resolve the situation. If the tissue feels stretchy, it may be reduced manually as explained in Chapter 5, on page 133.

The presenting part

- Is it a head? It is important to consider that the presenting part may not be a head; otherwise one risks missing an undiagnosed breech presentation. Exam findings with a frank breech may mimic those with an extremely malpositioned head: no sutures or fontanelles are felt and the leading part feels soft and spongy, as with a caput. One way to clarify this situation, short of ultrasound, is to do a sterile speculum examination. The presence of hair confirms a cephalic presentation.

- What is the fetal station? In relation to the imaginary transverse plane between the ischial spines, where is the leading edge of the bony skull? (Fig. 3.13)

- To assess station by vaginal examination:
  ○ Stations of descent are expressed in centimeters above or below the level of the ischial spines, which is designated as zero station. When the head has not yet entered the pelvis, the leading edge is said to be 'floating'.

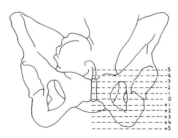

Fig. 3.13 Stations of descent.

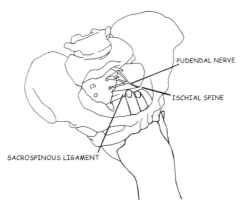

PUDENDAL NERVE

ISCHIAL SPINE

SACROSPINOUS LIGAMENT

3

Fig. 3.14 Finding the sacrospinous ligament.

- ○ The examiner first finds the approximate location of one ischial spine. It is easiest to do this by reaching with one's dominant hand diagonally across the mother's pelvis (so a right-handed provider will palpate the right maternal spine). On a woman with a normal midpelvis the spine will be blunt and not easily palpated, so approximating its location takes practice. It helps to find the sacrospinous ligament and follow it with two fingers from the midline to the place of insertion on the sidewall as shown in Fig. 3.14. Because this insertion point is also the location of the pudendal nerve, the mother may report an achy sensation when the examiner's fingers press there.
- ○ Second, the examiner compares the level of the leading edge of the head with the level of the ischial spines. It is imperative to use enough pressure to feel the bone, to avoid mistaking a large spongy caput for a head at a lower station.

- ● Consider assessing station abdominally
  According to the World Health Organization, 'When there is a significant degree of caput or moulding, assessment by abdominal palpation is more useful than assessment by vaginal exam[22]. Using abdominal palpation, an experienced clinician can:
  - ○ Assess descent with a minimum of intrusion
  - ○ Avoid the infection risks of a vaginal examination with ruptured membranes

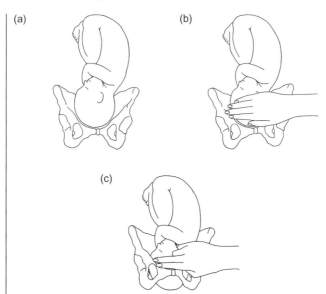

Fig. 3.15a (a) Fetal head above pubic symphysis; (b) Palpating fetal head at 5/5; (c) Palpating fetal head at 2/5. Adapted from WHO, 2003 reference 22.

○ Make more accurate assessments when considering the relative safety of cesarean surgery, operative vaginal delivery or watchful waiting in a given situation.

To assess descent by abdominal palpation, the examiner mentally divides the fetal head in five sections, each about the width of one of the examiner's fingers.

○ When the entire fetal head is above the pubic symphysis as in Fig. 3.15a, it can be palpated with all five fingers and is said to be 'five fifths' palpable (5/5). See Fig. 3.15b. (At this height, the head is mobile, or floating.)

○ When the head can only be felt with two fingers above the symphysis, it is said to be 'two fifths' palpable (2/5), or partially engaged, as shown in Fig. 3.15c.

○ When the head is entirely below the symphysis, it is said to be 'zero fifths' palpable (0/5), or deeply engaged.

○ A less precise measure, but one that is useful when learning to assess fetal descent, is how deeply the examiner's fingers are inserted before reaching the head[23]. Assuming average length fingers:

a. If the fetal head is floating, the fingers will be inserted completely into the vagina and not reach the leading edge of the head (Fig. 3.16a). If the fetal head is beginning to descend, but still above the ischial spines, the fingers, when inserted completely into the vagina, will be able to palpate the head with the tips of the fingers.

b. If the fetal head is at the level of the ischial spines, the fingers are inserted about half way before meeting the head (Fig. 3.16b).

c. At lower stations the fingers reach the head easily (Fig. 3.16c).

Assessment of station, like many other internal examinations in labor, is not precise and varies from examiner to examiner. In a

(a) Floating, or well above spines

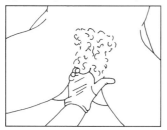

(b) At level of spines – O station

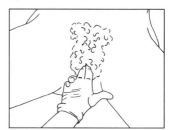

(c) Below the spines

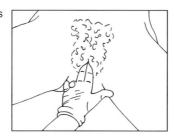

Fig. 3.16 a, b, and c Vaginal examinations to assess descent.

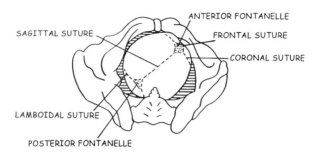

Fig. 3.17 Landmarks on the OP fetal head (sagittal suture in oblique diameter).

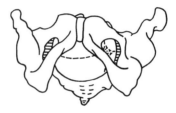

Fig. 3.18 Asynclitic fetus in occiput transverse.

slow second stage, progress may be incremental, in millimeters, rather than centimeters. When progress is in question, sequential evaluation by the same examiner is important.

A high station in active phase, especially in a nullipara, may suggest malposition or true cephalo-pelvic disproportion.

- Evaluating fetal position: using palpable landmarks of sutures and fontanelles, where is the occiput in relation to the maternal pelvis?
  - The first step is to find the most easily palpated landmark, the sagittal suture. Some degree of asynclitism is normal as the head comes into the pelvic brim in early labor. But with a well-positioned head, throughout most of labor the sagittal suture is usually in the right or left oblique diameter and roughly in the middle of the pelvis (Fig. 3.17). It may also be in a transverse diameter. During the second stage of labor when internal rotation normally occurs, it rotates 45–90° to the anterior-posterior diameter of the pelvis.

    If the sagittal suture is palpated just below the pubic arch, it indicates asynclitism (Fig. 3.18).

If the sagittal suture cannot be felt at all, there is probably significant asynclitism, usually posterior, with the posterior parietal bone, (that is the parietal bone next to the woman's back) leading and the sagittal suture tucked under the symphysis pubis.

○ Next the fontanelles are assessed by following the sagittal suture line in both directions from the midline. The posterior fontanelle is smaller and has three points. It does not actually

Table 3.2 Fetal positions viewed from below and from front of pelvis.

Position	Vaginal view	Front view of fetus in pelvis
LOA	Fig. 3.19a	Fig. 3.19b
ROP	Fig. 3.19c	Fig. 3.19d
LOT	Fig. 3.19e	Fig. 3.19f

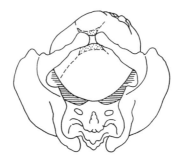

Fig. 3.20   Asynclitic fetus in right occiput posterior.

feel like a triangular space as much as the joining of three suture lines. The anterior fontanelle is much larger and has four points and is shaped like a diamond. See Table 3.2 and Fig. 3.17.

○   Even when it is not possible to accurately locate fontanelles, malposition can often be detected. It is important to notice whether the head fits more or less symmetrically. When the fetal head is malpositioned, it does not fill the pelvis. On examination, the head feels tight in the front of the pelvis, as if it is sitting over the pubic symphysis, while there is room in the back of the pelvis (Fig. 3.20).

Identifying fetal position is perhaps the single most difficult assessment to make during intrapartum vaginal examinations. Studies that have compared digital assessments of fetal position with ultrasound assessments concluded that digital assessment of position was often impossible, especially in the first stage[24], and when done, was accurate only 54% of the time when the occiput was posterior or lateral. During the first stage of labor, digital assessment of position was accurate only 31% of the time[25]. Therefore, for accuracy, a more comprehensive assessment of fetal position would have to be made, including Leopold's maneuvers, location of fetal heart tones, and other assessments, in addition to digital examinations. Ultrasound might also be utilized in situations where clinical assessments of fetal position are not done, but the information is desired.

Evaluating flexion of the fetal head

With a well-flexed head in the occiput anterior position, the small posterior fontanelle is palpable in the right or left oblique diameter of the pelvis, while the anterior fontanelle is not. When a large fontanelle is easily palpated, the fetus is usually in a posterior, deflexed position.

Evaluating presence of molding

Molding, the overlap of the bones of the head as a response to pressure during labor, permits the fetal head to better accommodate the tight fit through the maternal pelvis. Molding is often necessary for fetal descent. However, if excessive and occurring early in labor, molding may be a sign of difficulty[27]. Evaluating the degree of molding, together with the stage of labor, the station, estimated fetal size and other variables, can aid in the assessment of dysfunctional labor. Molding obscures fontanelles and makes sutures feel more prominent.

Evaluating caput

Caput formation, the accumulation of fluid in the tissue of the scalp, is also a result of pressure on the fetal head. It normally occurs in second stage labor with active descent, but may be present in active phase of the first stage with ruptured membranes. The finding of 'caput formation' with a high station could actually represent an undiagnosed breech (soft and spongy) rather than caput. It might also signify OP position or disproportion. Extensive caput also makes assessment of position and station more difficult, and is sometimes mistaken for descent. As the caput forms, the swelling expands lower in the pelvis, but the fetal head may not have descended at all.[26]

Evaluating the application of the head to the cervix

Is the head well applied to the cervix, or does the cervix feel like an 'empty sleeve'? With a malpositioned head, it is common to find that the cervix is soft and stretchy, but during contractions the head does not press against it. This gives the impression of a poor fit, rather than a 'rigid' cervix, as described on page 54.

The vagina and bony pelvis

- Do the vaginal muscles feel soft and stretchy, or tight and unyielding?
- Are there any obvious bony abnormalities, that is, flat sacrum, short diagonal conjugate, prominent ischial spines, narrow pubic arch or rigid, prominent coccyx, or does the pelvis feel generally normal?
- When all of these seem normal, it is reassuring to the careprovider.

Quality of contractions

Normal labor is characterized by uterine contractions that are involuntary and intermittent, and that increase in frequency, duration, and intensity over time. A contraction can be visualized as a bell-shaped curve consisting of three phases: the *increment*, as the intensity builds, the *acme* or peak, and the *decrement* or relaxation as the intensity diminishes.

Normal coordination of the myometrium during labor causes the uterus to differentiate into a thick, muscular upper segment and a thinning, stretchy lower segment. *Retraction*, the continual shortening of the vertical muscle fibers, is what enables the uterus to decrease intrauterine space, thus opening the cervix and pushing the fetus down and out.

When labor is dysfunctional, it is important to evaluate uterine activity. Poor uterine activity can be a primary cause of dysfunctional labor, or it may be an effect of some other problem, such as a malpositioned fetus[9]. The expression 'the uterus has a brain' aptly describes this interplay. When the fetus does not fit well through the pelvis, uterine contractions often diminish in response to this relative obstruction[28].

The following features of contractions should be assessed:

- *Frequency* is measured from the start of one contraction to the start of the next. Some providers note this as the number of minutes from onset to onset, that is, 'q five minutes'. Others record the number of contractions in a 10-minute period. Contractions of active labor are characterized by a frequency of 2–5 in ten minutes. Concerns arise when contractions are more frequent than five contractions in ten minutes (tachysystole). Because placental blood flow is markedly diminished during the most intense contractions of labor, a minimum rest of 30 seconds between contractions is essential to adequate fetal oxygenation. When there are more than five contractions in ten minutes, the fetus may not have adequate time between them to recover. This is rarely a problem in spontaneous labor but must be considered when labor is induced or augmented, particularly with misoprostol[29].

- *Duration* is assessed as the time from the start of a contraction to its end. This varies considerably depending on the stage or phase of labor. Early labor is characterized by contractions that may last only 20–30 seconds and active labor by contractions lasting 60–90 seconds.

- *Resting time* is calculated by subtracting the duration from the frequency. For example, if the contractions occur every three minutes and last 80 seconds, there is a 100 second rest from the end of one contraction until another contraction begins. Frequency, duration and resting time can be assessed using palpation, or measured objectively by electronic monitoring, using either a tocodynamometer (external, pressure-sensitive device) or an intrauterine pressure catheter.

- *Resting tone* is the degree to which the uterus relaxes between contractions. The normal resting tone in labor is less than 15 mm Hg. High resting tone is abnormal and potentially hazardous for both mother and fetus. It could lead to uterine dystocia and fetal distress, due to inadequate capillary refilling and oxygen transfer at the placental site. See below for ways to assess resting tone by palpation.

- *Intensity* is defined as the rise in intrauterine pressure above the resting tone with each contraction. Contractions capable of dilating the cervix are 30–50 mm Hg above resting tone at their acme. Contractions become even stronger in second stage and reach their maximum magnitude in the third stage, although third stage contractions are not perceived to be painful[30].

Although resting tone and intensity can be assessed with external palpation, precise measurements are only possible using an intrauterine pressure catheter. The external monitor's measurements of resting tone and intensity may depend on the placement of the tocodynamometer and therefore may be less reliable than palpation by an experienced examiner.

When one is not using external or internal electronic monitoring devices, the following methods to assess contractions are used:

- *External palpation.* Using a watch that displays seconds and firm pressure of the fingers on the fundus, the examiner assesses frequency, duration, and resting time. Resting tone and intensity can also be reasonably estimated. Between contractions, the fundus should feel soft and relaxed. The onset of the contraction may be palpated before the woman feels it. At the peak of an adequate contraction, the woman's fundus is not indentable and feels 'woody hard'. The examiner may detect the relaxation phase and the end of the contraction before the woman's pain sensation abates. This is because the woman is still perceiving the stimulation of nerve fibers in the cervix and lower uterine segment. One guide to aid the inexperienced practitioner in assessing uterine contraction intensity is the 'nose, chin, forehead' analogy. If the uterus feels like one's nose when pressed, the intensity is mild; like one's chin, it is moderate; like one's forehead, it is intense.

  Women with substantial adipose tissue over the uterine wall will be more difficult to assess, but with practice, the caregiver can learn to appreciate differences in contraction quality in these situations.

- *Internal assessment.* If the caregiver suspects that contractions are not intense enough to dilate the cervix, examining the cervix during a contraction can help evaluate contraction strength. This examination is much more uncomfortable for the woman than a cervical assessment done between contractions, so it is important to explain the rationale and obtain her permission. Then the caregiver gently inserts her/his fingers before the contraction begins, and holds the finger tips against the cervix. With the onset of a good contraction, the edges of the cervical os stretch, and the head descends, pressing against the cervix. If there is a forebag with intact membranes, it becomes tight and full. Inadequate contractions are not strong enough to produce these changes, and little stretch is palpated. The cervix may have the 'empty sleeve' feel because the head is not brought into contact with it.

- *Mother's perception.* Because pain perception is highly variable from woman to woman, this alone is a poor indicator of contraction quality. However, the mother is able to report whether contractions are becoming more intense over time, a feature of normally progressing active phase labor. Dysfunctional labor may be characterized by contractions becoming less frequent, lasting less time or feeling less intense.

ASSESSING THE MOTHER'S CONDITION

Trained clinicians assess many factors in a laboring woman's condition. This section addresses factors in the woman's condition that may influence labor progress. Progress may be positively or negatively affected by the degree to which the woman's physical and emotional well-being are attended to.

3

Hydration and nourishment

Page 21 discusses adverse effects of dehydration during labor. Women in labor also require approximately 50–100 kcals per hour to maintain adequate muscle function[31]. Research literature firmly supports the free use of oral intake (both fluids and solids) during labor[32]. Given access, some women will naturally take in the necessary calories and nutrients to sustain them during labor, but some may need to be reminded. Prolonged labor may be both a cause and an effect of dehydration and insufficient caloric intake. Therefore, the caregiver should focus on prevention. Having non-acidic, easy to digest carbohydrate snacks and drinks available (broth, electrolyte balanced sports drinks, fruit, honey, toast, etc.), and encouraging regular intake in small amounts at a time, is an effective strategy to prevent maternal exhaustion caused by dehydration and poor caloric intake.

Assessment of adequate hydration and nourishment include:

- *Urine.* The laboring woman should void at least every two hours and produce urine that is light in color. Dark, concentrated or scant urine suggests inadequate fluid intake.
- *Ketonuria.* Ketosis, the accumulation of ketones as a result of metabolizing stored fat in the absence of adequate carbohydrate availability, occurs normally in response to both exertion and fasting[32]. Controversy exists about whether the presence of ketone bodies in urine during labor is a sign of maternal compromise[31].
- *Temperature.* A slight rise in temperature is normal during labor, but if elevated more than one degree or so and labor has

been prolonged, it may signal dehydration. Significant increase in temperature (>38°C, 100.4°F), especially in the presence of ruptured membranes, may signal infection, a serious intrapartum complication.

- *Emesis.* Vomiting is common in labor. However, when it is prolonged or persistent, dehydration may result. Replacing fluids lost in this way requires additional intake, either oral or intravenous.
- *Fluid loss through perspiration.* Women laboring in warm conditions, especially those in warm water baths, need additional fluids. They should be encouraged to drink more often. Offering liquids after each contraction or two is preferable to asking if she wants a drink.
- *Maternal distress.* Women who become seriously compromised due to inadequate intake may feel anxious, exhausted and sick. Severe dehydration can exacerbate nausea and vomiting. Intravenous rehydration may be necessary.

Vital signs

During prolonged labor, maternal vital signs should be assessed at regular intervals between contractions. The presence of elevated blood pressure, pulse, or abnormal respiration rate must be noted and addressed. When maternal and fetal vital signs are normal, there is more leeway for patience.

Psychology

Much has been written about the adverse effects of psychological distress on the progress of labor[33-39].

The mother's psychology works synergistically with the physical parameters of labor. Poor labor progress can be caused by psychological distress, and psychological distress can be a result of a long and difficult labor. When there are no apparent physical reasons for poor labor progress, a psychological source should be considered.

The caregiver's ability to communicate with the woman is essential. Establishing a trusting and supportive relationship provides the foundation for positive communication. This is easier when there has been a prenatal relationship, but many skilled intrapartum caregivers are able to establish good rapport quickly with women they have never met before. Chapter 2 and others address the importance of minimizing psychological stress for laboring women. Chapter 8 includes information about creating a supportive labor environment, assessing a woman's emotional state and building trust through good communication.

ASSESSING THE FETUS

Most of the time, the term fetus of the otherwise healthy woman tolerates prolonged or dysfunctional labor well. When the information about fetal well-being is reassuring, caregivers and parents can focus on the challenges of coping with and resolving the dysfunction. Injecting a bit of humorous reassurance ('Your baby is enjoying this labor more than you are!') reminds the mother who is working hard in her labor that she has a healthy fetus who is not becoming compromised.

Conversely, when signs of fetal compromise are present, attention to resolving the distress becomes paramount. Most parents are keenly aware of the potential for fetal compromise during labor and appreciate accurate information from caregivers when concern about the baby arises. Elements of fetal assessment discussed here are the fetal heart rate, gestational age and the presence or absence of meconium in the amniotic fluid.

Fetal heart rate (FHR)

The primary source of information about fetal well-being during labor is the fetal heart rate and its response to contractions. For this reason, clinicians receive training and continuing education on interpreting fetal heart rate patterns. The relative benefits and risks of continuous electronic fetal monitoring (EFM) using external or internal instrumentation versus intermittent auscultation (IA) using a fetoscope or hand-held Doppler are summarized in Chapter 2.

This section provides an overview of intermittent auscultation. It is not meant to be a text on fetal surveillance, but rather, a learning tool for those who want to restore the use of auscultation for healthy, low-risk, pregnant women.

Intermittent auscultation is the method of fetal assessment used in home and free-standing birth center settings. In many hospitals, auscultation has been largely abandoned, although it is a reliable method of monitoring fetal well-being[9 and 40-42]. The technique is described here in detail.

How to perform intermittent auscultation

A handheld Doppler device or a fetal stethoscope may be used. Ultrasound detects motion of the heart valves and converts this into a manufactured sound that replicates the fetal heartbeat. The fetal stethoscope is specially designed to utilize the bone conduction of the examiner's skull to transmit the subtle sounds of fetal cardiac activity through the ear pieces. It generally requires more practice than the Doppler to use correctly.

The Doppler offers these advantages:

- Allows easier auscultation in a variety of maternal positions
- Allows auscultation during contractions
- Enables parents and others to hear the FHR
- Does not require pressure on the woman's abdomen, so is more comfortable
- Can be adapted for use in water (requires special waterproof probe)
- Compared to fetoscope, some studies showed improved neonatal outcome[42]

The fetoscope offers these advantages:

- Detects true sounds of fetal heart, including dysrhythmias, avoiding risks of artifact or detecting maternal pulse in error
- Provides no additional ultrasound exposure
- Requires no battery or mechanical parts that can malfunction
- Can also be used to help verify fetal position, as discussed earlier in this chapter

The following protocols are derived from published recommendations of the American College of Obstetricians and Gynecologists,[40] Association of Women's Health, Obstetric and Neonatal Nurses[44] and Society of Obstetricians and Gynecologists of Canada[41]. These organizations publish updated guidelines from time to time.

- *Frequency of auscultation.* Every 15–30 minutes in the first stage of labor, and every five minutes in the second stage or when the mother begins pushing. If an abnormality is detected, more frequent auscultation should be performed. There are no good data that confirm benefit from evaluating the fetal heart rate during the latent phase of labor.
- *Timing of auscultation.* Contractions should be palpated, and immediately following the contraction the fetal heart rate should be counted for 60 seconds. No research has confirmed the value of auscultating during a contraction.
- *Method of counting.* Various methods may be used. The 'six-second method' gives a quick approximation of the range of the FHR within a one minute period. Count the rate for six seconds and multiply by ten, wait four seconds and repeat this process 6–10 times. The maternal pulse should be evaluated periodically to ensure that the rate that is being counted is fetal and not maternal.

In 1997, a report from the US National Institute of Child Health and Human Development Research Planning was published establishing 'standardized and unambiguous definitions of fetal heart rate tracings'[45] as obtained from electronic fetal monitoring. Table 3.3a shows their definitions of these components of fetal heart rate interpretation, including which of these components can be evaluated using intermittent auscultation.

Table 3.3a

Baseline rate: the number of beats per minute (BPM) measured between contractions	
Assessed using EFM	Assessed using auscultation
By observing 10 minutes of a tracing (not necessarily continuous, but at least 2 minutes duration), and rounding to the nearest 5 BPM, excluding periodic changes which occur in response to contractions, fetal activity, marked variability, or segments that differ by more than 25 BPM.	Counting beats for one minute, between contractions. Normal baseline, as well as tachycardia and bradycardia can be assessed with auscultation.

Points to keep in mind:

- Normal baseline rate is 110–160 BPM in a term or post-term fetus, or 120–160 in a preterm fetus.
- Tachycardia is a baseline rate that exceeds 160 BPM (considered severe when greater than 180). When seen with decreased variability, prolonged or repetitive decelerations, meconium staining or maternal fever, tachycardia indicates fetal compromise.
- Bradycardia is a baseline rate that is less than 110 BPM, although a rate of 100–119 may be normal in the term or post-term fetus. If less than 100 BPM bradycardia is considered moderate, if less than 80 BPM, it is considered severe.
- Decreased variability as seen on EFM, may be due to fetal sleep, prematurity, or maternal medication. It may also be due to fetal compromise, especially if it is seen with other risk factors such as decelerations, abnormal baseline, meconium or maternal complications.

Table 3.3b

Baseline variability: Fluctuations in the baseline FHR which are characteristically irregular in frequency and amplitude of the heart beat from peak to trough of each beat	
Assessed using EFM	Assessed using auscultation
By *visual* assessment of an EFM tracing. Normal variability is an amplitude range of 6 to 25 BPM.	Cannot be assessed using intermittent auscultation, but may be *approximated* using the '6 second method' of counting over a minute's time.

Reassuring signs of fetal well-being that can be assessed without EFM

- Accelerations of the FHR with or without fetal scalp or vibro-acoustical stimulation[46] (See Table 3.3c)
- Normal baseline FHR without decelerations (See Table 3.3d)
- Absence of arrhythmia in the FHR

Table 3.3c

Accelerations: increases in the FHR above baseline; considered a sign of fetal well-being	
Assessed using EFM	Assessed using auscultation
By observing a monitor strip: ● Onset is abrupt, rising to the peak in less than 30 seconds. ● Acme is greater than 15 BPM above baseline. ● Duration is greater than 15 seconds and less than 2 minutes.	May be heard and documented[45]. However, specific duration and amplitude of acceleration requires EFM[42].

● Fetal movement reported by the woman or palpated by the examiner
● Clear amniotic fluid

A brief overview of gestational age, meconium, and indications for consultation is relevant.

Gestational age

Both preterm (less than 37 completed weeks) and post-term (greater than 42 completed weeks) fetuses are more vulnerable to the stress of labor.

With premature fetuses:

● Decelerations of the FHR are more ominous.
● Additional risk to the fetus may be related to the etiology of the preterm labor, that is, infection or placental abruption.

With post-term fetuses:

● There are increased risks of oligohydramnios, meconium passage, meconium aspiration syndrome and cord compression[14].
● There is increased likelihood of macrosomia, with its attendant labor risks (CPD and malposition)[8].

Table 3.3d

Decelerations: decreases in the FHR below baseline associated with contractions	
Assessed using EFM	Assessed using auscultation
By observing monitor strips one might see any of the following patterns: ● *Early decelerations* mirror the shape of the contraction, with gradual decrease (taking longer than 30 seconds from onset to nadir) in FHR and gradual return to baseline with the cessation of the contraction. These decelerations are thought to be primarily a vagal nerve response caused by head compression, and are benign. ● *Late decelerations* are gradual decreases in FHR reaching a nadir (which may be subtle, i.e. 10–30 BPM below baseline) *after* the peak of the contraction. In most cases the deceleration begins after the onset of the contraction, reaches its nadir after the peak of the contraction, and resolves after the contraction ends. These decelerations are thought to be a consequence of poor placental perfusion and, especially when seen with decreased variability and an absence of accelerations, are considered ominous. ● *Variable decelerations* are abrupt decreases in FHR (from onset of deceleration to nadir in less than 30 seconds), characterized by a deeper nadir (greater than 15 BPM) that returns to baseline more rapidly than the other types of decelerations (less than 2 minutes from onset to recovery) and occur with variable relationship to contractions. These decelerations are considered to be a consequence of cord compression, and are seen commonly. They are only of concern if they are persistent, becoming deeper than 70 BPM, or prolonged.	Decelerations may be heard with intermittent auscultation, but differentiating the three types of decelerations is only possible using EFM.

- Some studies have found a positive association between post-dates and shoulder dystocia. Other studies have not confirmed this association, except when there is macrosomia[47].
- There is increased risk for placental insufficiency, resulting in growth restriction and higher rates of stillbirth.

Meconium

The fetus may pass meconium in utero when there is a brief episode of hypoxia that causes relaxation of the anal sphincter. Meconium in the amniotic fluid during labor may indicate a compromise in fetal oxygenation. However, it is more often a normal maturational event, occurring more frequently as gestational age reaches and exceeds 40 weeks, and in 35–50% of all post-dates pregnancies[14].

Meconium should be considered a sign of fetal compromise if it is:

- Associated with a non-reassuring fetal heart rate pattern.
- Associated with maternal fever or other signs of infection.
- Thick, dark colored or particulate (containing discrete pieces or chunks).

Consultation

Midwives who attend births in out-of-hospital settings (home and birth centers) usually consider the following conditions to be indications for intrapartum consultation and/or transfer to a hospital[48–52].

- Non-reassuring FHR assessment.
- Gestational age less than 37 weeks.
- Gestational age greater than 42 weeks.
- Significant (dark, thick or particulate) meconium in the amniotic fluid.

PUTTING IT ALL TOGETHER

Assessing progress in first stage

As discussed in Chapter 2, clinicians and researchers use a variety of definitions of normal labor progress. In Chapter 4, we discuss some distinctions between pre-labor and latent phase contractions, with pre-labor characterized by contractions that do not change in quality or change the cervix over time. The latent phase is characterized by persistent contractions that do effect change, albeit slow and sometimes subtle. Active phase is defined as the time when contractions are more intense and frequent and the rate of change becomes more accelerated. With this in mind, different criteria should be used to assess labor progress for latent phase from the criteria for active phase.

Features of normal latent phase

- The cervix softens and effaces slowly but progressively.
- Fetal station may or may not change.
- Dilation is minimal, up to 3–4 cm.
- Contractions may be regular or irregular, with varying frequency and duration, but are usually mild to moderate in intensity.
- Normal duration is up to 20–24 hours. This is the longest phase of labor for most nulliparas[53].
- The woman may be distractable during contractions and carry on 'normal' activities between contractions.
- Mother does not become exhausted.

Features of normal active phase

- Cervical effacement becomes complete, later in multiparas than in nulliparas.
- The rate of cervical change increases over time, although progress may not be uniform from hour to hour.
- Dilation progresses over time to full dilation, but the rate of dilation varies tremendously between women.
- The fetal head engages, particularly in the nullipara.
- The fetal head descends to lower stations, especially toward the completion of first stage.
- The woman's behavior becomes serious and focused, both during and between contractions. Her coping behaviors may become more dramatic.
- If there is back pain, the place that hurts moves downward over time.
- Normal symptoms during rapid dilation may include an increase in bloody show, nausea, vomiting, shaking, irritability, anger, a desire to minimize stimulation or feelings of desperation.

- This phase lasts longer for nulliparas than for multiparas.
- The upper limit of normal duration varies from author to author (see Chapter 6).
- Mother and fetus fare well with the work of labor.

Assessing progress in second stage

There is often a latent phase after full dilation and before the fetus descends enough to trigger a pushing urge (see Chapter 7). If the active phase of second stage is defined to include full dilation *and spontaneous active pushing efforts*, active second stage progress is assessed by linear descent of the head and concludes with the birth of the baby.

3

Features of normal second stage

- The mother has spontaneous pushing urges (unless she has regional anesthesia).
- Contractions increase or remain strong and intense, though they may be shorter or less frequent than those in late first stage.
- The fetal head may mold and form a caput.
- All of the mechanisms of labor are accomplished: descent, flexion, internal rotation, birth of the head, restitution, external rotation, and birth of the shoulders and body of the fetus.
- Upper limits of normal duration vary, but are longer for nulliparas than for multiparas.
- The mother and the fetus fare well with pushing.

CONCLUSION

This chapter has covered methods of assessment of mother and fetus that are relevant to diagnosis and management of dystocia. These techniques enable the clinical care provider not only to identify dystocia, but also its specific etiology.

REFERENCES

1. ACOG (2003) Dystocia and the augmentation of labor. ACOG Practice Bulletin no. 45. American College of Obstetricians and Gynecologists. *Obstetrics and Gynecology*, 102, 1445–54.

2. Andrews, C., & Andrews, E. (1983) Nursing, maternal postures, and fetal position. *Nursing Research*, **32**, 336–41.

3. Sutton, J. (2001) *Let Birth Be Born Again: Rediscovering and Reclaiming Our Midwifery Heritage*. Birth Concepts, UK.

4. Scott, P. (2003) *Sit Up and Take Notice: Positioning Yourself for a Better Birth*. Great Scott Publications, Tauranga, New Zealand.

5. Tully, G. (2004) *Spinning Babies: Childbirth Made Easier with Fetal Positioning*. Maternity House Publishing, Bloomington, Minn.

6. Varney, H. (2003) *Varney's Midwifery*, 4th ed. Jones & Bartlett, Boston, Mass.

7. Gregory, K., Henry, O., Ramacone, E., Chan, L. & Platt, L. (1998) Maternal and infant complications in high and normal weight infants by method of delivery. *Obstetrics and Gynecology*, **92**, 503–513.

8. ACOG (2000) Fetal Macrosomia. ACOG Practice Bulletin no. 22. American College of Obstetricians and Gynecologists. *Obstetrics and Gynecology*, **98**, 1–11.

9. Enkin, M., Keirse M., Neilson, J. *et al.* (2000) *A Guide to Effective Care in Pregnancy and Childbirth*, 3rd edn. Oxford University Press, Oxford.

10. Baum, J., Gussman, D. & Wirth, J. (2002) Clinical and patient estimation of fetal weight vs. ultrasound estimation. *Journal of Reproductive Medicine*, **47**, 194–8.

11. Nahum, G. (2002) Predicting fetal weight. Are Leopold's maneuvers still worth teaching medical students and house staff? *Journal of Reproductive Medicine*, **47**, 752–60.

12. Levine, A., Lockwood, C., Brown, B., Lapinski, R. & Berkowitz, R. (1992) Sonographic diagnosis of the large for gestational age fetus at term: does it make a difference? *Obstetrics and Gynecology*, **79**, 55–8.

13. Nahum, G. & Stanislaw, H. (2002) Validation of a birth weight prediction equation based on maternal characteristics. *Journal of Reproductive Medicine*, Sept. **47**, 752–760.

14. Gabbe, S., Niebyl, J. & Simpson, J. (2002) *Obstetrics: Normal and Abnormal Pregnancies*, 4th edn. Churchhill Livingstone, New York.

15. Olah, K. & Gee, H. (1992) The prevention of preterm delivery – can we afford to continue to ignore the cervix? *British Journal of Obstetrics and Gynaecology*, **99**, 278–80.

16. Olah, K., Gee, H. & Brown, J. (1993) Cervical contractions: the response of the cervix to oxytocin stimulation in the latent phase of labour. *British Journal of Obstetrics and Gynaecology*, **100**, 635–40.

17. Granstrom, L., Ekman, G. & Malmstrom, A. (1991) Insufficient remodelling of the uterine connective tissue in women with protracted labour. *British Journal of Obstetrics and Gynaecology*, Dec. **98**, 1212–116.

18. Bishop, E. (1964). Pelvic scoring for elective induction. *Obstetrics and Gynecology*, 24, 267.

19. Peisner, D. & Rossen, M. (1985) Latent phase of labor in normal patients: a reassessment. *Obstetrics and Gynecology*, **66**, 544–648.
20. Neumann, Y. (2004) Doing a pelvic exam with a woman who has experienced sexual abuse, Chapter 12. in: *When Survivors Give Birth* (eds P. Simkin & P. Klaus). Classic Day Publishing, Seattle.
21. Holcomb, W. & Smeltzer, J. (1991) Cervical effacement: variation in belief among clinicians. *Obstetrics and Gynecology*, **78**, 43–5.
22. Publication Department of Reproductive Health and Research (2003) *Managing Complications in Pregnancy and Childbirth: A Guide for Midwives and Doctors*, p. 82, World Health Organization, Geneva.
23. Flint, C. (1986) *Sensitive Midwifery*. Heinemann Nursing, Oxford.
24. Akmal, S., Kametas, N., Tsoi, E., Hargreaves, C. & Nicolaides, K. (2003) Comparison of transvaginal digital examination with intrapartum sonography to determine fetal head position before instrument delivery. *Ultrasound Obstetrics and Gynecology*, **21**, 437–40.
25. Souka, A., Haritos, T., Basayiannis, K., Noikokyri, N. & Antasaklis, A. (2003) Intrapartum ultrasound for the examination of the fetal head position in normal and obstructed labor. *Journal of Maternal Fetal Neonatal Medicine*, **13**, 59–63.
26. Oxorn, H. (1986) *Human Labor and Birth*, 5th edn. McGraw-Hill, New York.
27. Bennett, V. & Brown, L. (1999) *Myles Textbook for Midwives*, 13th edn. Churchill Livingstone, London.
28. Neilson, J., Lavender, T., Quenby, S. & Wray, S. (2003) Obstructed labour. *British Medical Bulletin*, **67**, 191–204.
29. Crane, J., Young, D., Butt, K., Bennett, K. & Hutchens, D. (2001) Excessive uterine activity accompanying induced labor. *Obstetrics and Gynecology*, **97**, 926–31.
30. Whitely, N. (1975) Uterine contractile physiology: applications in nursing care and patient teaching. *Journal of Obstetrical, Gynecological and Neonatal Nursing*, **4**, 54–8.
31. Sinclair, C. (2004) *A Midwives Handbook*. Saunders, St Louis.
32. Ludka, L. & Roberts, C. (1993) Eating and drinking in labor: a literature review. *Journal of Nurse-Midwifery*, **38**, 199–207.
33. Odent, M. (1992) *The Nature of Birth and Breastfeeding*. Bergin & Garvey, Westport, Conn.
34. Odent, M. (1999) Birth reborn, Chapter 6. In: *The Scientification of Love*. Free Association Books, London.
35. Lederman, R., Lederman, E., Work, B. & McCann, D. (1981) Relationship of psychological factors in pregnancy to progress in labor. *Nursing Research*, **25**, 94–8.
36. Lederman, E., Lederman, R., Work, B. & McCann, D. (1981) Maternal psychological and physiologic correlates of fetal-newborn health status. *American Journal of Obstetrics and Gynecology*, **139**, 956–60.

3

37. Wuitchik, M., Bakal, D. & Lipshitz, J. (1989) The clinical significance of pain and cognitive activity in latent labor. *Obstetrics and Gynecology*, **73**, 35–42.

38. Simkin, P. (2002) Supportive care during labor: a guide for busy nurses. *Journal of Obstetrical, Gynecological and Neonatal Nursing*, **31**, 721–32.

39. Simkin, P. & Klaus, P. (2004) *When Survivors Give Birth: Understanding and Healing the Effects of Early Sexual Abuse on Childbearing Women.* Classic Day Publishing, Seattle.

40. ACOG (1995) Intrapartum fetal heart rate patterns: monitoring, interpretation and management. *ACOG Technical Bulletin* no. 218. 1–9. American College of Obstetricians and Gynecologists, Washington, DC.

41. Liston, R., Crane, J. & the SOGC Fetal Health Surveillance Working Group (2002) Fetal Health Surveillance in Labour. *Clinical Practice Guidelines* 112: 1–13. Society of Obstetricians and Gynecologists of Canada, Ottawa.

42. Royal College of Obstetricians and Gynaecologists (2001) *The Use of Electronic Fetal Monitoring. The Use and Interpretation of Cardiotocography in Intrapartum Fetal Surveillance.* (Evidence-based clinical guidelines; no. 8). Royal College of Obstetricians and Gynaecologists Press, London.

43. Goodwin, L. (2000) Intermittent auscultation of the fetal heart rate: a review of general principles. *Journal of Perinatal Neonatal Nursing*, **14**, 53–61.

44. AWHONN (1997) *Fetal Heart Monitoring Principles and Practices.* Association of Women's Health, Obstetric and Neonatal Nurses, Washington, DC.

45. NICHHD (1997) Electronic fetal heart rate monitoring: Research guidelines for interpretation. National Institute of Child Health and Human Development Research Planning Workshop. *American Journal of Obstetricians and Gynecology*, **177**, 1385–90.

46. Paine, L., Johnsen, T., Turher, M. & Payton, R. (1986) Auscultated fetal heart rate accelerations, Part II. An alternative to the non-stress test. *Journal of Nurse-Midwifery*, **31**, 73–77.

47. Lewis, D., Edwards, M., Asrat, T., Adair, C., Brooks, G. & London, S. (1998) Can shoulder dystocia be predicted? *Journal of Reproductive Medicine*, **43** (8), 654–8.

48. College of Midwives of British Columbia (1997) *Standards of Practice and Indications for Discussion; Consultation and Transfer of Care.* College of Midwives of British Columbia, Vancouver.

49. National Health Insurance Board of the Netherlands (2000) Final Report of the Obstetric Working Group of the National Health Insurance Board of the Netherlands. *Obstetric Manual.* National Health Insurance Board of the Netherlands.

50. MAWS (2002) *Indications for Consultations in an Out-of-Hospital Midwifery Practice.* Midwives' Association of Washington State, Seattle, Washington.

51. TMA (2001) *Practice Guidelines*. Tennessee Midwives' Association, Memphis.
52. MMA (1998) *Transfer Criteria*. Massachusetts Midwives Alliance, Stoneham, Mass.
53. Friedman, E. (1978) *Labor: Clinical Evaluation and Management*, 2nd edn. Appleton Century Crofts, New York.

3

Chapter 4

Prolonged Pre-Labor and Latent First Stage

Is it dystocia? 82
When is a woman in labor? 83
Preventing the occiput posterior (OP): measures to use before labor, 84
The woman who has hours of contractions without dilation, 87
The six ways to progress in labor, 87
Support measures for women who are at home in pre-labor and latent phase, 89
Some reasons for excessive pain and duration of pre-labor or latent phase, 91
Iatrogenic factors, 91
Cervical factors, 92
Fetal factors, 92
Emotional factors, 92
Troubleshooting measures for painful prolonged pre-labor or latent phase, 93
Measures to alleviate painful irregular non-dilating contractions in pre-labor or latent phase, 95
Synclitism and asynclitism, 95
Conclusion, 101
References, 101

IS IT DYSTOCIA?

A diagnosis of dystocia is usually based on the rate of labor progress, which, one might expect, would depend on the time of the onset of labor. Ironically, diagnosing the onset of labor, as fundamental as it may seem, is not easy, and wide disagreement exists among experts on how to decide when labor begins.

When is a woman in labor?

Two obstetricians whose teachings have dominated Western obstetrics for half a century, represent the extremes of opinion regarding the definition of labor. Emmanuel Friedman defined labor as follows:

'The onset of labor is defined simply as that time at which the patient first perceived regular uterine contractions. There is no way to distinguish true labor from false except by hindsight (when the contractions cease or when active dilation begins).'[1]

This definition is used today[2-3]. At the other end of the spectrum, Kieran O'Driscoll and his colleagues in Ireland use a very precise definition of labor: painful contractions occurring at least every ten minutes or closer, accompanied by at least one of the following: bloody mucous vaginal discharge; spontaneous rupture of the membranes; or complete cervical effacement[4]. A woman may have regular painful uterine contractions for many hours or even days before meeting O'Driscoll's criteria for labor.

These widely varying definitions of labor result in different management styles. According to Friedman, the latent phase in nulliparas averages nine hours, and is considered 'prolonged' at 20 hours. O'Driscoll and colleagues would deny that a woman in Friedman's 'latent phase' is even in labor unless she exhibits the other signs and symptoms mentioned above. Friedman suggested drug-induced rest for women with a prolonged latent phase, whereas O'Driscoll and colleagues do not admit her to the hospital or acknowledge any clinical significance to these contractions, regardless of what the women feel and think.

In this book, our definition of labor is based on distinguishing between progressing and non-progressing contractions. Progressing contractions increase in one or more of the following measures: intensity, duration, and frequency. Non-progressing contractions remain the same over time. We define pre-labor as a period of regular, non-progressing contractions, without an increase in cervical dilation, which may or may not continue without interruption into the latent phase. We define the latent phase of labor as the period beginning with continuous progressing contractions accompanied by cervical effacement and dilation and ending at 3 to 4 cm. When the onset of labor is spontaneous, the woman or her partner is the informant regarding the time of onset. They should be taught to time her contractions and to differentiate between progressing and non-progressing contractions.

Using a definition of labor based on more specific characteristics than Friedman's 'regular contractions' recognizes that 'false' or pre-labor contractions can be differentiated from true labor as they occur, not only in retrospect. This may aid the caregiver as he or she considers management options. It is important to recognize that from the woman's point of view, continuing contractions must be dealt with, whether or not they are becoming more frequent, intense, or longer, or are accompanied by bloody show or ruptured membranes. Pre-labor must not be discounted; nor, however, should it be treated as labor.

Preventing the occiput posterior (OP): measures to use before labor

Chapter 3 describes methods to assess fetal position before labor. Estimates of OP at the onset of labor range between 10 and 20%, and at delivery, 5%[5]. If an OP position is diagnosed before labor, what can be done to facilitate rotation to an occiput transverse (OT) or occiput anterior (OA) position? What can be done to maintain the OA position once it is achieved? First of all, spontaneous rotation, without intervention, occurs in most labors, though this rotation is often accompanied by greater discomfort and prolonged labor. One study found that 87% of fetuses who were OP at the onset of labor rotated to OA by delivery; but 68% of fetuses who were OP at delivery had been OA at the onset of labor and rotated to OP during labor[5]. In other words, of 100 fetuses, 20 are OP at the onset of labor, but only 2 of those would still be OP at delivery. The other 3 fetuses who are OP at delivery would have begun labor in the OA position. Factors that cause rotation from OA to OP during labor may include the shape and size of both the fetal head and maternal pelvis, but also maternal position during labor[6-8]. Other factors, such as the use of epidural analgesia and the woman's bearing-down efforts, are discussed in Chapters 5 and 6.

The concept of 'Optimal Fetal Positioning', originally described by Sutton and Scott[6-8], refers to maternal positions that can be used over the last weeks of pregnancy to improve the likelihood of the fetus being in the left occiput anterior or transverse (LOA or LOT) position at the onset of labor, which is optimal for comfort and progress during labor. They also describe ways to encourage or maintain an LOA position during labor, which will be discussed in Chapter 5.

Sutton and Scott advocate that the woman spends very little time during late pregnancy in supine or semi-reclining positions, which encourage an OP fetal position. Rather, she should spend most of her time in forward-leaning positions, such as those seen in Figs 4.1 a–d: sitting up straight on a birth ball or straight chair; sitting and leaning forward on a table or desk (keeping her knees lower than her hips); hands and knees (doing pelvic rocks, also known as the 'cat-cow' movement in yoga); the open knee-chest position; kneeling and leaning forward onto a chair seat, beanbag, or birth ball; or standing and leaning forward on a table or counter; lying down to rest or sleep in a semi-prone position on her left side. Sutton and Scott state that such postures utilize gravity and also increase the space at the pelvic brim, within the pelvis, and at the outlet. They advocate exercise, such as walking, swimming in a prone position, and yoga, while discouraging squatting, and long car trips sitting in a bucket seat.

Though frequently recommended, the hands and knees position, with pelvic rocking or abdominal stroking, to turn OP or OT fetuses during late pregnancy has been evaluated in only two randomized controlled trials[9–10], and the findings of the two were opposite. In one trial, including 100 women with OP or OT fetal positions, one or two ten-minute periods in a hands and knees position with or without pelvic rocking, abdominal stroking, or both, was more likely to result in an OA fetal position in the short term, when compared to a sitting position[9].

The other randomized controlled trial included 2547 women with unknown fetal positions. It compared incidence of OP position at birth in two groups of women: the experimental group, who, beginning at 37 weeks' gestation, spent two ten-minute periods per day in a hands and knees position combined with pelvic rocking; and the control group, who took a daily walk. They found no differences between groups in the incidence of OP at birth[10]. The lifestyle changes promoted by Sutton and Scott have never been studied with randomized controlled trials.

Despite the lack of supporting evidence, the concept of Optimal Fetal Positioning is widely accepted, especially by midwives and their clients, who are willing to try the positions during late pregnancy in

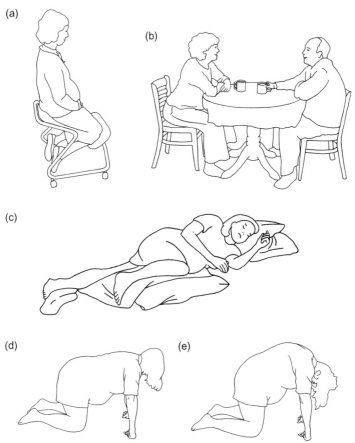

Fig. 4.1 Helpful positions for later pregnancy: (a) Sitting straight.
(b) Sitting leaning forward. (c) Semi-prone on left side. (d and e) Doing
the pelvic rocking exercise ('cat-cow' in yoga).

hopes of averting one of the most troublesome deterrents to normal
progress and vaginal birth.

Because fetuses in OA or OT sometimes rotate to OP during labor[5],
techniques to maintain an OA or rotate OT and OP fetuses to OA

during labor should be learned and used by caregiving staff. These are described later in this chapter and in the next two chapters.

The woman who has hours of contractions without dilation

Sometimes it takes many hours, even days, of contractions before a woman's cervix dilates to 3 or 4 cm. To a great extent, the duration of pre-labor (sometimes referred to as 'false labor') or of latent first stage depends on the state of her cervix at the onset of contractions. The more unripe, uneffaced, and posterior her cervix, the greater the likelihood that her pre-labor or latent phase will last longer than it would with a more favorable cervix.

Despite the differences in definitions of labor, most obstetric and midwifery textbook authors seem to agree that very little should be done to try to speed either pre-labor or the latent phase of labor in the absence of medical problems requiring imminent delivery[1,4,11 and 12]. Because most slow-starting labors eventually resolve into normal labor patterns, a diagnosis of dystocia or dysfunctional labor cannot accurately be made before the active phase[1 and 13] (that is, in a nullipara before 3 to 4 cm dilated and nearly 100% effaced; in a multipara, before 4 to 5 cm dilated and 70 to 80% effaced). Special supportive measures, in addition to those listed in Chapter 1, may be used to help the woman through the time it takes for her cervix to change. Chart 4.1 illustrates a step-by-step approach to the problem of a prolonged pre-labor or latent phase. Some of these same supportive measures apply when a woman is undergoing cervical ripening and induction of labor, which may take place over several days.

In this section we suggest ways to assess and meet the woman's support needs during a prolonged pre-labor or latent phase, especially when she describes or appears to experience more pain than women usually report at this degree of cervical dilation.

THE SIX WAYS TO PROGRESS IN LABOR

Contractions without dilation are discouraging to the woman, who believes she is not making progress. She needs to understand that significant dilation can occur only when the cervix has already undergone preparatory changes. The caregiver should explain the reasons for pre-dilation (pre-labor) contractions in the context of the

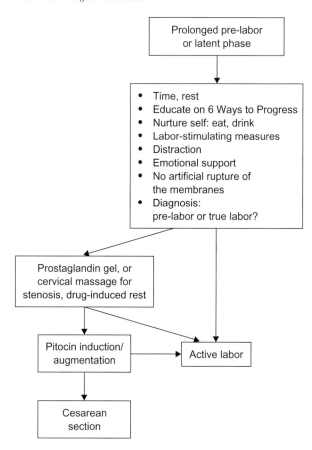

Chart 4.1   Prolonged pre-labor or latent phase.

Six Ways to Progress. Although health care providers know these six ways, they often ignore the fact that when the cervix has not undergone the first three steps (ripening, effacement, and anterior movement), significant dilation (beyond 3 cm in the nullipara, more in the multipara) rarely occurs. There is a tendency among caregivers to minimize the importance of these three cervical changes when, in fact, progress in those areas is a very good sign and a necessary precursor to dilation. If such progress is ignored, an incorrect diagnosis of dysfunctional labor may be made before the woman is even in labor.

The following six steps must be accomplished in order for a baby to be born vaginally. For most women, the first three steps take place gradually, simultaneously, and almost unnoticed over a period of weeks before labor begins. For a minority of women, however, hours or days of non-progressing pre-labor contractions are necessary to ready the cervix for dilation. Sometimes these contractions are intense enough to prevent sleep and the woman becomes discouraged and exhausted.

Here are the six ways to progress:

(1) The cervix moves from a posterior to an anterior position
(2) The cervix ripens or softens
(3) The cervix effaces
(4) The cervix dilates
(5) The fetal head rotates, flexes, and molds
(6) The fetus descends, rotates further, and is born.

4

If the woman's cervix is not yet dilating, even though she is having contractions, she will need reassurance from her caregiver that these pre-labor contractions are accomplishing the important job of preparing her cervix to dilate. She is making necessary progress. Before dilation begins, support measures should focus on educating the woman about the six ways to progress, encouraging her to engage in distracting activities, helping her to accept the slow progress of early labor as a normal variation, preventing exhaustion, meeting her nutritional needs, and keeping her comfortable.

Rotation, flexion, molding, and descent of the fetal head take place in active labor and second stage. These will be discussed in Chapters 5 and 6.

SUPPORT MEASURES FOR WOMEN WHO ARE AT HOME IN PRE-LABOR AND LATENT PHASE

While most women remain at home during this phase, some will come to the hospital and some will call for phone advice. It helps if they have been taught in advance or given a list of ways to cope with early labor. In the absence of medical contraindications, these suggestions will help the woman maintain normal progress and confidence:

- She should continue normal activities: rest (even if she cannot sleep) at night, do pleasant distracting activities during the day, for as long as possible, but avoid over-exertion.

- She should have her partner, a friend, a relative or a doula remain with her.

- If it is night time and the woman can rest, she should lie down or relax in the tub. (Please note: immersion in water in early labor may temporarily stop contractions and give the woman some rest[14–17]. This is an advantage if she needs rest, but may be a disadvantage if conditions exist that make it important that her labor progresses, e.g., prolonged pregnancy or prolonged rupture of membranes.)

- If she is unable to rest, or it is daytime, she should try distraction measures, such as:
  - going for a walk or having someone take her for a drive
  - visiting with friends or family
  - going to a movie or other entertainment, shopping
  - reading aloud to each other
  - preparing meals for after the birth, or baking bread
  - preparing the baby's clothing, bedding
  - watching videotapes, TV
  - doing a 'project', sorting photos, writing in a journal, cleaning a closet, drawing or painting
  - playing games, and others

- She should eat when hungry, unless she knows she is having a cesarean section (e.g. because of a herpes lesion, a complicated presentation, or other pre-existing condition). Best choices are easily digested complex carbohydrates (starchy foods, fruits, and vegetables). She should avoid greasy or highly spiced foods.

- She should drink to thirst. Water, broth, fruit juice, caffeine-free teas, or electrolyte-balanced beverages are good choices.

- She should begin using labor coping techniques during her contractions when distraction is no longer possible and she cannot walk through or talk through her contractions without pausing at the peaks. Such techniques as relaxation and self-calming, slow breathing (sighing), and attention-focusing are appropriate at this time.

- She should periodically time four or five consecutive contractions for duration, frequency, and interval to determine if her contractions are progressing. She should be given guidelines on when to come to the hospital (including guidelines on ruptured membranes).

- Some women, having no idea of what to expect from early labor, 'over-react', that is, they are preoccupied with every contraction, and they may rush to use learned coping techniques that are more appropriate for active labor. They often expect to be 5 or 6 cm dilated when they are first checked and are crushed when they are examined and found to be only 1 to 2 cm. They do not see how they are going to cope with the more intense contractions to come. A woman in this situation needs a chance to express her disappointment. The caregiver can help by acknowledging her disappointment, giving her some suggestions to reduce the intensity of the contractions, and proceeding to calm and relax her. She 'will need help to get her head back where her cervix is'[18].

4

If a woman arrives at the hospital earlier than necessary, she is often encouraged to return home. The manner in which this is handled can make her feel either more confident, knowledgeable, and willing to go home, or ashamed and angry, or afraid to leave the hospital. If the above support measures are followed, the former is more likely.

SOME REASONS FOR EXCESSIVE PAIN AND DURATION OF PRE-LABOR OR LATENT PHASE

For some women, pre-labor or latent phase is extremely painful and prolonged for a variety of reasons:

Iatrogenic factors

Oxytocin-induced contractions are sometimes painful and debilitating, especially when the cervix is unripe, or when the woman's contractions come every two or three minutes and her cervix is only 1 or 2 cm dilated.

There may be policies or practices that restrict the woman to bed. Reasons for such a policy include ruptured membranes (see page 94);

continuous electronic fetal monitoring (see pages 23–31); pregnancy-induced hypertension (see page 94). In many cases, restriction to bed is not required, but no one encourages the woman to get out of bed.

Cervical factors

An unripe cervix at term may indicate insufficient remodeling of the connective tissue, which causes cervical resistance[19–20] to increasing intrauterine pressures, or the presence of muscle fibers in the cervix[21], which cause cervical contractions during uterine contractions.

A scarred or fibrous cervix, possibly from previous surgery (e.g. cauterization, cryosurgery, cone biopsy[11], or other causes) may increase the resistance of the cervix to effacement and the first few centimeters of dilation. Contractions of great intensity for many hours or days may be required to overcome this resistance, after which dilation often proceeds normally.

Fetal factors

These include: occiput posterior position of the fetus, or brow, face presentation, or large, unengaged fetal head.

Emotional factors

Extreme fear, anxiety, loneliness, stress, or anger may lead to a build-up of catecholamines and a resulting slowdown in progress (see pages 17–18). Women who are unsupported emotionally, or have experienced previous difficult childbirths, traumatic experiences such as physical or sexual abuse, substance abuse, multiple hospitalizations, or domestic violence may find early labor unexpectedly painful.

Exhaustion, discouragement, and feelings of hopelessness result from a long pre-labor or latent phase. The woman's optimism and coping ability diminish and her pain worsens as time goes on without apparent progress.

It may be helpful to ask the woman about her emotional state during latent labor. Her answer may assist the caregiver in diagnosing emotional distress. Between contractions, questions such as 'what was going through your mind during that contraction?' or 'how are you feeling right now?' or 'why do you think this labor is going slowly right now?' may reveal that the mother is distressed or worried over specific concerns. Knowing these concerns will help the caregiver support the woman emotionally. See Chapter 8, pages 265–268, for more on how to help an emotionally distressed woman.

Women having painful non-progressing pre- or early labors often appear to be much further along in labor than they are. The contractions may be so intense that they must rely on coping strategies that others might not use until late in the first stage. Of course, they also become discouraged and hopeless. It is important that caregivers do not label the woman as being frail or unable to cope, or discount or minimize the woman's pain at this early stage of labor. It does not help her cope and only results in her feeling unsupported.

The next section offers suggestions to improve labor progress or reduce discomfort in early labor. Of course, if fetal distress, macrosomia, malpresentation, inadequate contractions, or other complications are diagnosed, the supportive measures will have to be tailored to the situation.

TROUBLESHOOTING MEASURES FOR PAINFUL PROLONGED PRE-LABOR OR LATENT PHASE

- Follow the general measures for early labor as described in Chapter 2.

- For the pain and discouragement that may accompany some labor inductions or an unripe or scarred cervix, reassure the woman that under these circumstances early labor is more challenging, but it does not necessarily mean that active labor will be abnormal[19].

  Such women also need validation, intense emotional support and physical comfort. Try not to contribute to her self-doubt or worries by suggesting that something is wrong.

- If she is discouraged over slow dilation or non-progressing contractions, remind the woman that before her cervix can dilate, it must move forward, ripen, and efface – each of which is a positive sign of progress. Be sure to disclose any progress in these areas to her whenever you check her cervix. See Six Ways to Progress on pages 87–89.

- Avoid the term 'false labor' because it implies that her contractions are somehow 'unreal' and that because her cervix is not dilating, the contractions are not accomplishing anything significant. Such implications are most discouraging to the woman who is experiencing them. In fact, if her cervix is changing at all, these pre-labor contractions are preparing the cervix for dilation.

- Encourage her to seek and use those positions or movements that she finds more comfortable. See Monitoring the mobile woman's fetus, pages 23–30, for suggestions on monitoring during induced labor.

- Offer a bath, shower or massage as a temporary relaxer and pain reliever.

- Transcutaneous electrical nerve stimulation (TENS) may be especially useful to relieve back pain during early labor. TENS is more useful for back pain than for other labor pain and is more beneficial when introduced early in labor. See Chapter 8.

- A drug-induced rest with a pain reliever may be an appropriate choice. *Note*: If at all possible, do not restrict the woman to bed. Before restricting a woman with ruptured membranes to bed (which is a requirement in many hospitals even if the fetal head is engaged) the caregiver might auscultate the fetal heart and assess fetal movement with the woman in an upright position. Sometimes the upright position actually protects against a prolapsed cord, as gravity may keep the head applied to the cervix, thus preventing the cord from slipping through.

- Many caregivers, especially in North America, restrict the woman with pregnancy-induced hypertension to bed in late pregnancy and in labor, because blood pressure is usually lowered while a woman lies on her left side. Whether such treatment has resulted in improved outcomes or less progression of pre-eclampsia is not known[22]. The topic has received too little study to draw conclusions. However, if you are caring for a woman who is in bed with pregnancy-induced hypertension, you can explain why left-sided bedrest is being asked of her (while acknowledging the lack of study in this area). Help her focus on comfort measures that she can use while in bed. Relaxation, breathing patterns, vocalization, guided imagery, visualizations, other attention-focusing measures, and massage of her back or feet may help. In addition, if limited walking is acceptable, she may walk to and from the bathroom, to use the shower or tub (both of which frequently lower high blood pressure). Having some choices regarding her position boosts her morale.

- Assess the woman's emotional state during early labor and, if she is distressed, try appropriate measures to help improve her emotional state. See the Toolkit, Chapter 8, pages 265–268.

- For exhaustion, discouragement, and hopelessness, you can raise her spirits by suggesting a change: have her wash her face, comb her hair, brush her teeth, take a walk, play some upbeat music. These measures are especially effective as the sun comes up after a long night with little progress. The new day can renew spirits.

- Have a good talk with her and her partner, encouraging them to express their feelings. Acknowledge and validate their feelings of frustration, discouragement, fatigue, or even anger at the staff for not 'doing something' to correct the problem. She may benefit from a good cry, followed by a pep talk and perhaps a visit from a friend or family member who is rested and optimistic.

MEASURES TO ALLEVIATE PAINFUL IRREGULAR NON-DILATING CONTRACTIONS IN PRE-LABOR OR LATENT PHASE

4

If early contractions are painful and irregular with little or no progress in dilation, it makes sense to consider persistent asynclitism or another unfavorable fetal position, such as occiput posterior (Fig. 4.2).

Synclitism and asynclitism

Labor normally begins with the fetal head in asynclitism (the head is angled so that one of the parietal bones, rather than the vertex, presents at the pelvic inlet as shown in Fig. 4.3a and b). This facilitates passage of the fetal head through the pelvic inlet, and then the head usually shifts into synclitism (Fig. 4.4) so that the vertex presents as the head descends further. However, sometimes the asynclitism persists and, if so, it can keep the fetus from rotating and descending[23]. Without descent, the head may not be well applied to the cervix and contractions often become irregular and ineffective. At this stage of labor, it is difficult or impossible (and not considered very clinically important) to assess the angle and position of the fetal head. However, if contractions are irregular and ineffective for a long time, position changes and movements may correct the problem and improve the contraction pattern.

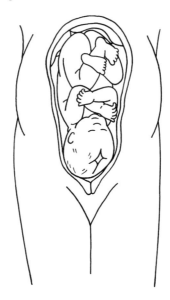

4

Fig. 4.2　Right occiput posterior, abdominal view.

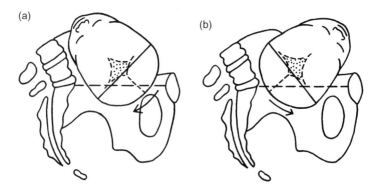

Fig. 4.3　(a) Posterior asynclitism. (b) Anterior asynclitism.

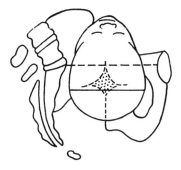

Fig. 4.4 Synclitism.

If the woman is having her first baby or has good abdominal muscle tone, having her lean forward often moves the fetus' center of gravity forward, encouraging its head to pivot into a more favorable position (Figs 4.5–4.7). This may evenly disperse or increase the head-to-cervix force, leading to more regular, more effective contractions. If the woman's abdominal muscle tone is poor and her abdomen is pendulous, the fetus' center of gravity may fall so far forward that the fetus is not well-aligned with the pelvic inlet. She might benefit from a semi-reclining position (Fig. 4.8). Having her 'lean back' in this way may move the fetus' center of gravity toward her back, thus allowing the head to put more pressure on the cervix during the contractions, and may lead to more regular, more effective contractions.

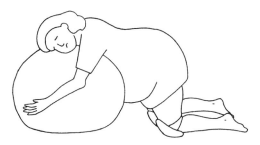

Fig. 4.5 Kneeling with a ball and knee pads to correct possible posterior asynclitism.

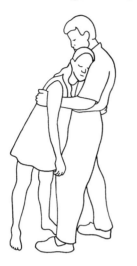

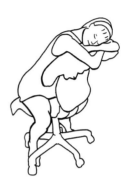

Fig. 4.6 Standing, leaning forward on partner.

Fig. 4.7 Straddling a chair.

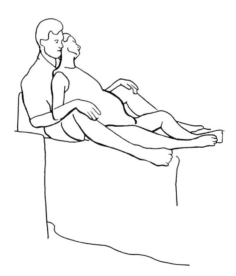

Fig. 4.8 Semi-sitting.

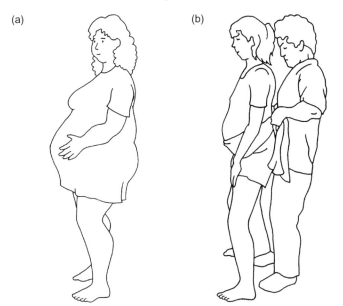

Fig. 4.9 (a) Abdominal lifting. (b) Abdominal lifting with a shawl.

King suggests abdominal lifting (Fig. 4.9a and b) with a pelvic tilt during contractions at any time in labor if the woman has back pain in association with pendulous abdominal muscles, a short waist, a previous back injury, or an occiput posterior baby[24]. Abdominal lifting, when it works well, realigns the angle between the baby's torso and the pelvic inlet. The contractions then become more efficient in pressing the baby's head onto the cervix. See Toolkit, Chapter 7, pages 239–241 for specific instructions. We suggest that fetal heart tones be checked periodically by the nurse or midwife during a contraction with abdominal lifting. In the remote possibility that the heart rate decelerates, it might be due to anterior placement of the umbilical cord. If so, the pressure on the low abdomen could compress the cord, and abdominal lifting should not be used.

The open knee–chest position may take advantage of gravity to allow the fetus to 'back out' of the woman's pelvis, rotate, and descend again in a more favorable position.

El Halta[25], an American midwife, teaches the open knee–chest position for specific symptoms in pre-labor or the latent phase, when there is a long period of frequent, irregular and brief uterine contractions, usually accompanied by severe persistent backache, but resulting in little or no dilation. El Halta's experience is that such a contraction pattern is associated with an occiput posterior position. She instructs the woman to spend 30 to 45 minutes in an open knee–chest position, that is, her hips are flexed to an angle greater than 90° (Fig. 4.10).

The open knee–chest position tilts the pelvis forward with the inlet lower than the outlet. This allows gravity to encourage the unengaged

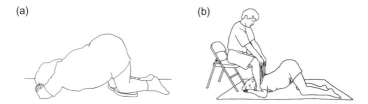

Fig. 4.10 (a) Open knee–chest position. (b) Open knee–chest position, shoulders resting on partner's shins.

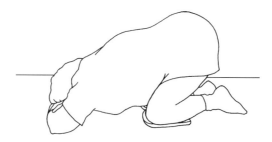

Fig. 4.11 Closed knee–chest position with knee pads. Pressure of thighs on abdomen may interfere with fetal rotation.

OP fetal head out of the pelvis, and may allow the head to reposition more favorably toward OA before re-entering the pelvis. By contrast, a 'closed knee–chest position' (Fig. 4.11) would mean that the woman's hips and knees are flexed so that her thighs are beneath her abdomen and the pelvic inlet is higher than the outlet. This gives less room for the fetus to move out of the pelvis and less gravity effect.

CONCLUSION

Prolonged pre-labor and the latent phase of labor in themselves rarely indicate a complication, although they are discouraging and exhausting for the woman. Suggestions are given for coping with the discouragement, and early measures are described to correct possible fetal malposition. Most of the measures suggested here are well tolerated or favored by women, but if a woman finds them distressing or uncomfortable, she should be encouraged to do what she finds most helpful.

4

REFERENCES

1. Friedman, E.A. (1993) Dysfunctional labor. In: *Management of Labor* (eds W.R. Cohen & E.A. Friedman). p. 17. University Park Press, Baltimore.
2. Sinclair, C. (2004) *A Midwife's Handbook*. Saunders, St Louis, Missouri.
3. MacKenzie, S. (2004) Obstetrics: labor, Chapter 14. In: *University of Iowa Family Practice Handbook*, 4th edn. University of Iowa, Iowa City.
4. O'Driscoll, K., Meagher, D. & Boylan, P. (1993) *Active Management of Labour*, 3rd edn. Baillière Tindall, London.
5. Gardberg, M., Laakkonen, E. & Salevaara, M. (1998) Intrapartum sonography and persistent occiput posterior position: a study of 408 deliveries. *Obstetrics and Gynecology*, **91**, 746–9.
6. Sutton, J. & Scott, P. (1996) *Understanding and Teaching Optimal Foetal Positioning*. Birth Concepts, Tauranga, NZ.
7. Sutton, J. (2001) *Let Birth Be Born Again: Rediscovering and Reclaiming Our Midwifery Heritage*. Birth Concepts, UK, Bedfont, UK.
8. Scott, P. (2003) *Sit Up and Take Notice! Positioning Yourself for a Better Birth*. Great Scott Publications, Tauranga, New Zealand.
9. Andrews, C. & Andrews, E. (1983) Nursing, maternal postures, and fetal position. *Nursing Research*, **32**, 336–41.
10. Kariminia, A., Chamberlain, M., Keogh, J. & Shea, A. (2004) Randomised controlled trial of effect of hands and knees posturing on

incidence of occiput posterior position at birth. *British Medical Journal*, doi:10.1136/bmj.37942.594456.44 (26 January), 1–5.

11. Davis, E. (1997) *Heart and Hands: A Midwife's Guide to Pregnancy and Birth*, 3rd edn. Celestial Arts, Berkeley.

12. Varney, H. (1997) *Varney's Midwifery*, 3rd edn. Jones and Bartlett Publishers, Boston.

13. Fraser, W., Krauss, I., Boulvain, M., *et al.* (1995) Dystocia. Society of Obstetricians and Gynecologists of Canada (SOGC) *Clinical Guidelines*, **40**, 1–16.

14. Eriksson, M., Mattsson, L.A. & Ladfors, L. (1997) Early or late bath during the first stage of labour: a randomized study of 200 women. *Midwifery*, **13** (3), 146–8.

15. Odent, M. (1997) Can water immersion stop labor? *Journal of Nurse–Midwifery*, **42**, 414–16.

16. Simkin, P. & O'Hara, M. (2002) Nonpharmacologic relief of pain during labor: systematic reviews of five methods. *American Journal of Obstetrics and Gynecology*, **186**, S139–59.

17. Simkin, P. & Bolding, A. (2004) Update on non-pharmacological approaches to relieve pain and prevent suffering during labor. *Journal of Midwifery and Womens Health*, **49**, 489–504.

18. Wilf, R. (1980) Personal communication.

19. Olah, K. (1991) Measurement of the cervical response to uterine activity in labour and observations on the mechanism of cervical effacement. *Journal of Perinatal Medicine* **19** (Suppl 2), 245.

20. Olah, K., Gee, H. & Brown, J. (1993) Cervical contractions: the response of the cervix to oxytocic stimulation in the latent phase of labour. *British Journal of Obstetrics and Gynaecology*, **100**, 635–640.

21. Olah, K. & Neilson, J. (1994) Failure to progress in the management of labour. *British Journal of Obstetrics and Gynaecology*, **101**, 1–3.

22. Enkin, M., Keirse, M., Neilson, J. *et al.* (2000) Hypertension in pregnancy, Chapter 15. In: *A Guide to Effective Care in Pregnancy and Childbirth*, 3rd edn. Oxford University Press, Oxford.

23. Oxorn, H. (1986) *Human Labour and Birth*, 5th edn. Appleton Century Crofts, New York.

24. King, J.M. (1993) *Back Labor No More!! What Every Woman Should Know Before Labor*. Plenary Systems, Dallas.

25. El Halta, V. (1995) Posterior labor: a pain in the back. *Midwifery Today*, **36**, 19–21.

Chapter 5

Prolonged Active Phase of Labor

What is prolonged active labor? 104
Characteristics of prolonged active labor, 105
Possible causes of prolonged active labor, 106
Fetal and feto-pelvic factors, 108
Why fetal malpositions delay labor progress, 110
Artificial rupture of the membranes (AROM) with a malpositioned fetus, 111
Specific measures to address and correct problems associated with malposition, cephalo-pelvic disproportion and macrosomia, 112
Maternal positions and movements for suspected malposition, cephalo-pelvic disproportion, or macrosomia in active labor, 112
Forward-leaning positions, 114
Side-lying positions, 116
Asymmetrical positions and movements, 118
Abdominal lifting, 120
An uncontrollable premature urge to push, 120
If contractions are inadequate, 123
Immobility, 123
Medication, 125
Dehydration, 126
Exhaustion, 126
Uterine lactic acidosis as a cause of inadequate contractions, 127
When the cause of inadequate contractions is unknown, 128
If there is a persistent cervical lip or a swollen cervix, 131
Position changes to reduce an anterior lip or a swollen cervix, 132
Other methods, 132
Manual reduction of a persistent cervical lip, 133
If emotional dystocia is suspected, 134
Assessing the woman's coping, 134
Indicators of emotional dystocia during active labor, 136
Predisposing factors for emotional dystocia, 136

5

Helping the woman state her fears, 137
How to help a laboring woman in distress, 138
Special needs of childhood abuse survivors, 140
Incompatibility or poor relationship with staff, 141
If the source of the woman's anxiety cannot be identified, 142
Conclusion, 142
References, 143

WHAT IS PROLONGED ACTIVE LABOR?

The active phase of labor (or active labor) usually refers to cervical dilation greater than 3 cm accompanied by progressing contractions, that is, contractions that are becoming longer, stronger, and more frequent. It should be noted that multiparas sometimes reach 3, 4 or even 5 cm of dilation with only sporadic or non-progressing contractions. If a caregiver is unaware that a woman has been at 4 or 5 cms dilation for several days and does not review her contraction pattern, he or she may assume incorrectly that the woman is in labor. Then, once the woman is admitted to the hospital, if she makes no further progress and her contractions seem inadequate, the caregiver may diagnose her with 'failure to progress', when, in fact, she was never in labor. This illustrates why both dilation and the contraction pattern are crucial to a correct diagnosis of labor. A woman is not in labor until she begins having progressing contractions and her cervix dilates further.

The term 'prolonged active labor' refers to an insufficient rate of dilation after active labor has been diagnosed. The diagnosis of 'insufficient rate of progress' varies among authors: less than 1 cm per hour for at least two hours after labor progress has been established[1]; less than 1.2 cm per hour in a primigravida and less than 1.5 cm per hour in a multipara[2]; longer than 12 hours from 4 cm to complete dilation (which translates to 0.5 cm per hour)[3-4]. Zhang and colleagues noted that the criteria used today for diagnosis of protraction and arrest disorders in nulliparous women (largely derived from Friedman's work 30 to 50 years ago) are too stringent, and that women who give birth safely per vagina may progress at a rate of less than 0.5 cm per hour between 3 and 7 cm, and less than 1 cm per hour from 7 to 10 cm dilation[5].

CHARACTERISTICS OF PROLONGED ACTIVE LABOR

- The contractions slow down, that is, they become less intense, shorter in duration, and/or less frequent.
- Contractions take on a quality of sameness, neither progressing nor slowing down.
- The woman continues coping in the same way for hours, or finds labor easier to manage than it was previously.
- On a vaginal exam, the cervix is unchanged.

Clinical management of prolonged active labor varies, depending on the caregiver's philosophy and the woman's wishes, for example:

- One very common approach, once the diagnosis has been made, is to rupture the membranes (if that has not already been done) and start incremental doses of intravenous oxytocin. If these measures are unsuccessful in stimulating progress, a cesarean delivery is performed[6].

- In the active management of labor protocol[1], as practiced at the National Maternity Hospital in Dublin and elsewhere, the membranes are ruptured as soon as labor is diagnosed. If dilation is less than 1 cm per hour for two hours at any time after labor is diagnosed (regardless of cervical dilation), high doses of oxytocin are administered incrementally until a rate of at least 1 cm per hour is achieved.

- With midwifery care or a low intervention model of maternity care, the caregiver assesses the rate of dilation, but perceives a slow rate of dilation in the active phase as an indication for evaluation rather than medical intervention. The midwife or other low intervention caregiver is likely to make broader allowances for individual variations in progress of dilation, taking into account fetal and maternal tolerance of the delay and assessing signs of progress other than dilation, such as rotation of the fetal head, which is often a necessary precursor to further progress. (See Chapter 4, pages 87–89, Six Ways to Progress in Labor.) Such an approach relies on preventive measures, and time, patience, support, and primary interventions such as those offered in this book. The goals are to support the woman through the delay and

5

encourage labor progress[3,6–7]. Oxytocin and artificial rupture of the membranes are reserved for later use if necessary.

POSSIBLE CAUSES OF PROLONGED ACTIVE LABOR

Slowing or arrest of dilation in the active phase may sometimes be prevented or corrected by first using simple, low-cost interventions that carry little or no known risk. If they are not successful, then the woman will need the more powerful and complex obstetric interventions that are also more expensive and associated with more potential risks. Chart 5.1 illustrates a step-by-step approach to the problem of a prolonged active phase of labor.

The choice of intervention depends on the apparent cause of the problem. Causes of prolonged active labor include the following:

- *Fetal and feto-pelvic factors*: cephalo-pelvic disproportion (CPD) is a poor fit between the fetal head and maternal pelvis. CPD may involve a large head or a malpositioned head, in which the malposition (i.e. occiput posterior, occiput transverse, or asynclitism) causes the presentation of a larger diameter (e.g. a deflexed head) than when the vertex presents in an occiput anterior position. CPD may also occur with a discrepancy between the shape of the fetal head and the dimensions and shape of the maternal pelvis[8]. A persistently high station in the presence of adequate contractions may indicate a poor fit of the head, but not necessarily too large a head, within the pelvis.

- *Uterine factors*: inadequate intensity of contractions, uterine inertia.

- *Cervical factors*: persistent cervical lip, rigid os.

- *Emotional factors*: fear, anxiety, tension, or hostility. See Chapter 2.

- *Iatrogenic factors*: dehydration; restriction of movement; pain medications, epidural analgesia; inappropriate or excessive use of oxytocin.

- *Maternal factors*: exhaustion; short waist; lumbar lordosis, combined with lack of lumbar mobility; pendulous abdomen[9].

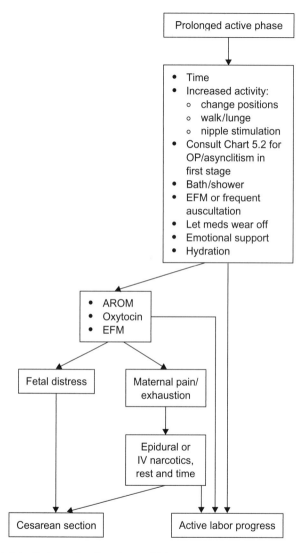

Chart 5.1 Prolonged active phase of labor.

- *Combination of etiologies or unknown etiology*: sometimes the delay in progress results from a combination of the above, for example a persistent malposition associated with a large baby, maternal fear or exhaustion, and inadequate contractions. Sometimes the cause is unclear. In such cases, the contractions appear adequate, fetal position appears favorable, fetal size seems average, and the woman appears to be coping well, but progress in dilation is slow. Patience, and trial and error, using a number of the measures discussed in this chapter, may result in greater progress without anyone figuring out exactly what the problem was. For example, a subtle undetectable variation in position or another problem may be corrected with the passage of time and a variety of movements and comfort measures.

Fetal and feto-pelvic factors

Malposition, macrosomia and cephalo-pelvic disproportion (CPD)

With information gained from observations of abdominal shape, abdominal palpation, location of fetal heart tones, the woman's symptoms, the contraction pattern, internal examination of the suture lines of the fetal skull, and/or ultrasound examination, the caregiver might suspect fetal malposition, macrosomia, or cephalo-pelvic disproportion (CPD). Even if the specific etiology is not clear, however, the primary interventions for all of these conditions are very similar, so a trial and error approach is usually acceptable. These interventions are grouped in this section.

Persistent asynclitism

At the onset of labor, most fetuses are in an asynclitic occiput transverse (OT) or occiput anterior (OA) position. This means the fetal head is angled so that one parietal bone enters the pelvis first, and the fetal biparietal diameter is not parallel to the plane of the inlet of the pelvis (Figs 5.1 and 5.2).

With contractions, the head usually pivots into synclitism, so that the fetal biparietal diameter is parallel to the plane of the inlet as it descends (Fig. 5.3). Only if asynclitism is persistent, that is, *remaining when the fetus is at a low station*, does it slow labor progress.

5

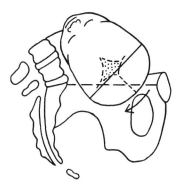

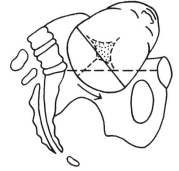

Fig. 5.1 Posterior asynclitism.   **Fig. 5.2** Anterior asynclitism.

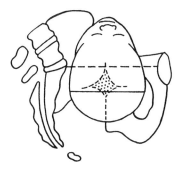

Fig. 5.3 Synclitism.

Occiput posterior

Estimates of the incidence of occiput posterior (OP) position at the onset of labor range between 10 and 20%, of all labors. OP is more common in primigravidas[10–11]. (See Chapter 3, pages 36–48 for ways to identify an OP fetus before the onset of labor.) Many fetuses who are occiput anterior (OA) at the onset of labor rotate to OP during labor, and most fetuses who are OP at the onset, rotate to OA spontaneously by late first stage or by delivery, and are born without difficulty. The latter is a common scenario for women with anthropoid pelves[11]. In the end, approximately 5% of fetuses are OP at

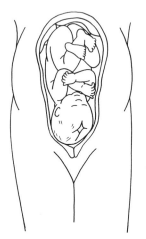
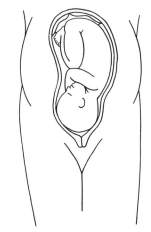

Fig. 5.4 Right occiput posterior, abdominal view.

Fig. 5.5 Left occiput anterior, abdominal view.

delivery[11–14], many of whom had been OA or OT at 8 cm or later[15]. Contractions, gravity, resilience of the muscles in the pelvis, shape of the pelvis, the woman's position and movement, fetal efforts, and other forces combine to cause rotation of the fetal head.

If they persist, OP (Fig. 5.4) and occiput transverse (OT) (Fig. 5.5) positions and asynclitism usually become problematic, with increased chances of operative delivery. If the woman's pelvis is roomy enough, however, time, support, and specific measures by the woman and staff will usually allow a vaginal birth. As long as the fetus and woman can tolerate them, these measures are often all that is necessary to solve the problem. But, if the problem persists in spite of these measures, that helps confirm the diagnosis of protracted or arrested active labor. At this time obstetric interventions are instituted.

Why fetal malpositions delay labor progress

When rotation or improved alignment is needed, it makes sense that labor will take more time than when the fetus is ideally positioned.

Dilation may begin later or take longer because the pressure of the fetal head or forewaters on the cervix, which normally enhances dilation, may be uneven or generally reduced. Descent may also be delayed until the fetal head rotates, flexes, or aligns with the plane of the pelvis.

One should always suspect a malposition, asynclitism, cephalo-pelvic disproportion, or macrosomia if:

- There is premature rupture of membranes at term[14]
- Contractions are irregular (varying in intensity and duration in an unpredictable way)
- Contractions 'couple' (two or three close together, followed by a relatively long interval)
- Contractions 'space out' or slow down in active labor
- The woman complains of back pain that may or may not go away between contractions
- Progress plateaus in active labor
- The woman has an uncontrollable urge to push long before dilation is complete

Artificial rupture of the membranes (AROM) with a malpositioned fetus

When there is a delay in active labor, caregivers often rupture the membranes to speed it up. There is some concern over the wisdom of such a practice when the fetus is malpositioned. Only a few small randomized controlled trials have been conducted on the use of amniotomy (with or without oxytocin) to augment progress in prolonged labor. Reviews of these trials by Hofmeyr[14] and Fraser[16] concluded that with mild delays in labor progress, amniotomy has not been clearly shown to be of greater benefit than conservative approaches to this problem. Trials comparing groups of women with arrested progress who were given amniotomy with women not given amniotomy found that amniotomy resulted in reduction of labor duration by approximately one hour, but no reduction in cesarean delivery and an increase in chorioamnionitis[17]. No trials have investigated the efficacy of amniotomy specifically in cases in which the fetus was known to be malpositioned.

If a fetal malposition, as opposed to other complications (such as inadequate contractions) slows labor progress, it raises questions about the wisdom of rupturing the membranes. When the fetus is poorly positioned, intact forewaters may provide some protection and maneuvering space for the fetal head. When the forewaters are removed, the malpositioned fetus may be subjected to uneven head compression, excessive molding, more pronounced caput succedaneum and a greater likelihood of operative delivery than would otherwise occur. Caldeyro-Barcia and colleagues raised these concerns years ago[18], and Sutton, a midwife who specializes in the prevention and correction of the OP position, suggests that rotation to OA is more difficult after membranes rupture[8]. Trials of amniotomy in OP labors are warranted to establish whether the malposition is more or less likely to self-correct with or without intact membranes. Without clear evidence of benefit, these potential risks (as well as other known risks of amniotomy – prolapsed cord and infection) remain a concern. It is surprising that the almost standard practice of performing amniotomy to augment slow labors associated with fetal malposition has not been adequately studied[14 and 16].

Specific measures to address and correct problems associated with malposition, cephalo-pelvic disproportion, and macrosomia

Besides those discussed here, see Chapter 1 for general measures to aid labor progress. As well as having her try a variety of positions (illustrated in this section), helping the woman to deal with back pain, which seems to be a common problem with fetal malposition, is an important element in her care. Baths and showers, back pressure and massage, the knee press, kneeling and swaying on the birth ball, transcutaneous electrical nerve stimulation, cold or warm compresses, and intradermal sterile water injections are effective in relieving back pain. These are described in Chapter 8.

MATERNAL POSITIONS AND MOVEMENTS FOR SUSPECTED MALPOSITION, CEPHALO-PELVIC DISPROPORTION, OR MACROSOMIA IN ACTIVE LABOR

Chart 5.2 illustrates a step-by-step approach to be used when an occiput posterior position or asynclitism is suspected.

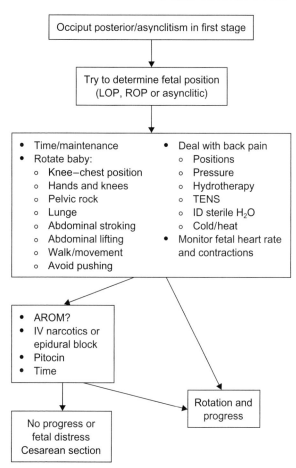

Chart 5.2 Suspected fetal malposition.

Maternal positions and movements alter the forces of gravity, pelvic dimensions[19–20], and the various pressures within the uterus and on pelvic joints. The position of the fetus is influenced by these changing forces. (See Chapter 7 for more information on each position and movement.)

Forward-leaning positions

Forward leaning positions (Figs 5.6a–j) may help reposition the fetus. These positions are vigorously promoted by Sutton[8] and Scott[21], and others, for their contributions to optimal fetal position. See Chapter 7 for an explanation of how these positions may correct some problems of a 'poor fit' between fetus and maternal pelvis.

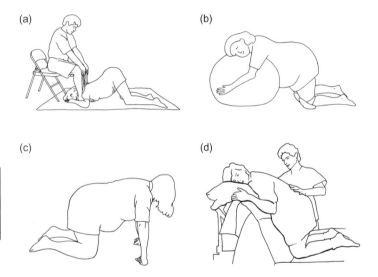

Fig. 5.6   Forward-leaning positions: (a) Open knee–chest position, resting shoulders on partner's shins. (b) Kneeling with a ball and knee pads. (c) Hands and knees. (d) Kneeling over bed back. (e) Kneeling, with partner support. (f) Kneeling on bed with partner support and knee pads. (g) Standing, leaning on bed. (h) Standing, leaning forward on partner. (i) Straddling a toilet, facing backward. (j) Straddling a chair.

(e)

(f)

(g)

(h)

(i)

(j)

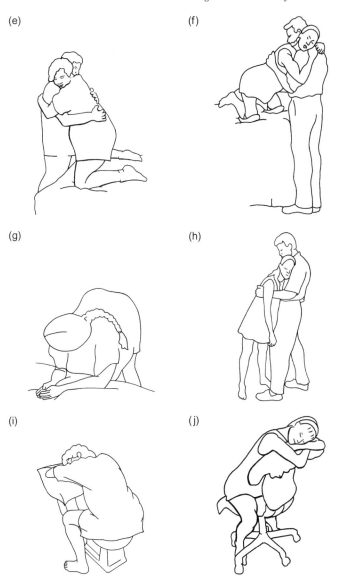

Fig. 5.6   (continued)

Side-lying positions for a *malpositioned fetus*

The effects of gravity on the fetus are quite different when a woman is in a pure side-lying versus a semi-prone (Sims') position. When the fetus is thought to be occiput posterior (OP):

- The woman using 'pure side-lying' should lie on the side toward which the occiput is already directed, with the baby's back 'toward the bed' (Figs 5.7 and 5.8). This encourages the OP baby to OT.
- If the woman is semi-prone, she should lie on the side opposite the direction of the occiput, with the fetal back 'toward the ceiling' (Fig. 5.9)[22].

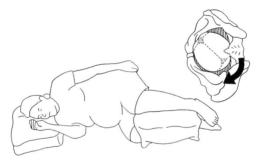

Fig. 5.7 Woman with an OP fetus in pure side-lying on the 'correct' side, with fetal back 'toward the bed'. If fetus is ROP, woman lies on her right side. Gravity pulls fetal occiput and trunk towards ROT.

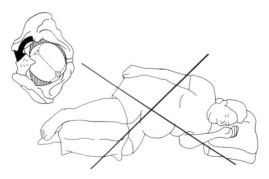

Fig. 5.8 Woman with an OP fetus in pure side-lying on the 'wrong' (left) side for an *ROP* fetus. Fetal back is toward the ceiling. Gravity pulls fetal occiput and trunk toward direct OP.

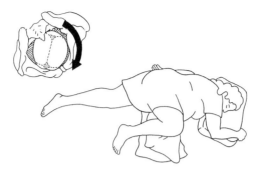

Fig. 5.9 Woman with an OP fetus in semi-prone on the 'correct' side, with fetal back 'toward the ceiling'. If fetus is ROP, the semi-prone woman lies on her left side. Gravity pulls fetal occiput and trunk toward ROT, then ROA.

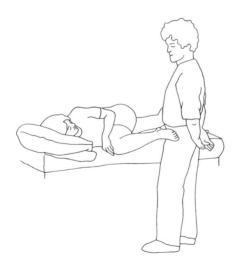

Fig. 5.10 Side-lying lunge.

With the 'side-lying lunge' (Fig. 5.10) steady pressure is applied to the sole of the woman's upper foot in the direction of her head, in order to increase hip flexion and abduction. This widens the pelvis, improving the chances of fetal rotation.

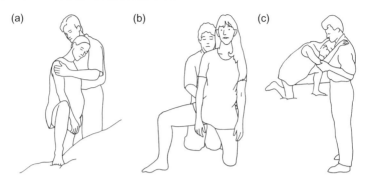

Fig. 5.11 (a) Standing with one leg elevated. (b) Asymmetrical kneeling. (c) Asymmetrical kneeling with partner support.

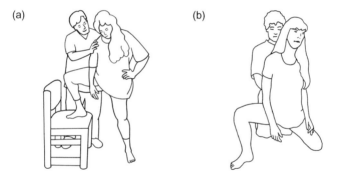

Fig. 5.12 (a) Standing lunge. (b) Kneeling lunge.

Asymmetrical positions and movements

Asymmetrical positions and movements, such as those pictured here (Fig. 5.11a–c), enlarge the pelvis on the side where the leg is raised, and slightly alter the internal shape of the pelvis. This may allow more space where it is needed for rotation. The lunge (Fig. 5.12a and b) uses weight-bearing and mild stretching of the hip abductors to create leverage to widen one side of the pelvis. To master the technique of the lunge, please see the instructions in Chapter 7, page 233, before teaching it to the woman in labor.

Note regarding supine and semi-sitting positions for occiput posterior

When a woman is fully supine or semi-sitting, gravity encourages the trunk of the OP fetus to lie next to the woman's spine, increasing the chances of supine hypotension, but also minimizing the likelihood of rotation to OA. These positions also increase the pressure of the fetal occiput against the woman's sacrum, thus worsening her back pain (Fig. 5.13a). There is a much greater likelihood of rotation, and less back pain when the woman sits upright or leans forward (Fig. 5.13b)[8,23].

When a woman is supine, the head of an occiput posterior fetus is directed more toward the pubic bone during contractions (Fig. 5.13c). When the woman is upright, the uterus, tilting forward, directs the fetal head into the pelvic basin (Fig. 5.13d).

(a)   (b)

(c)   (d)

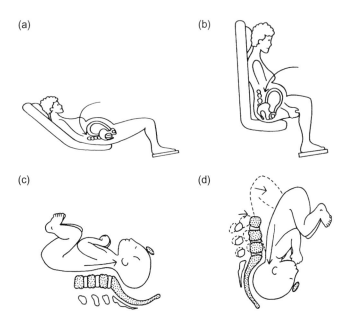

Fig. 5.13 (a) Woman reclining. Weight of uterus rests on her spine. (b) Woman upright. Fundus tilts forward. (c) Woman reclining. Head of OP fetus directed toward pubic bone. (d) Woman upright. Head directed into pelvic basin. Adapted from reference 23.

Abdominal lifting

To improve the alignment of the fetal trunk and head with the axis of the birth canal, the woman places her hands beneath her abdomen and during contractions lifts her abdomen while tilting her pelvis by bending her knees[9] (Fig. 5.14a and b). The use of a shawl (woven cloth measuring approximately 45 cm wide by 150–180 cm long) aids abdominal lifting. Caution: because the umbilical cord is sometimes located low and in front, there is a small possibility that it would be compressed with abdominal lifting. It is wise for the midwife or nurse to check the fetal heart rate occasionally during contractions while abdominal lifting is being done. If decelerations occur, abdominal lifting should be discontinued. See Chapter 7, page 239, for complete instructions on abdominal lifting.

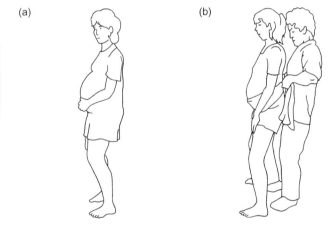

(a)   (b)

Fig. 5.14 (a) Abdominal lifting. (b) Abdominal lifting with a shawl.

An uncontrollable premature urge to push

An uncontrollable, almost convulsive urge to push during active labor sometimes accompanies an OP position, especially when the fetus is deeply engaged. The caregiver is faced with the question of whether the woman should push or not (Chart 5.3). On the one hand, with a prolonged active phase and an OP fetus, her pushing might lead to a swollen cervix or even a torn cervix, and no further progress. On the other hand, it is sometimes impossible for the woman to control this urge.

A change of position to hands and knees (Fig. 5.15a and b), semi-prone (exaggerated Sims, Fig. 5.16) or open knee–chest (Fig. 5.17a and b), may relieve the urge to push by using gravity to move the head away from the cervix and ease pressure on the posterior vaginal wall (which seems to be the factor responsible for the urge to push). Manual repositioning of the fetal head (page 170) may also help.

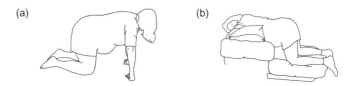

Fig. 5.15 (a) Hands and knees. (b) Kneeling on foot of bed.

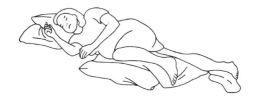

Fig. 5.16 Semi-prone (exaggerated Sims position).

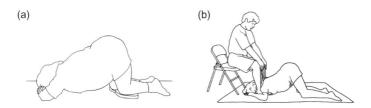

Fig. 5.17 (a) Open knee–chest position. (b) Open knee–chest position, shoulders resting on partners shins.

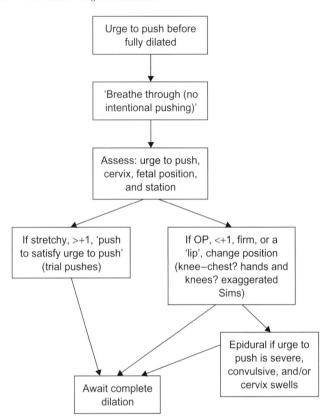

Chart 5.3   Premature urge to push.

IF CONTRACTIONS ARE INADEQUATE

If contractions seem to be inadequate in intensity, frequency and/or duration, consider whether immobility, medication, dehydration, or emotional factors could be contributing factors.

Immobility

Has the woman been in one position for over half an hour? Changing her position may trigger stronger contractions, either by shifting the fetus' weight or by improving circulation to the uterus. Upright positions and movements, including walking, may intensify contractions. The supine position, by contrast, is correlated with weaker contractions, when compared with other positions[24-25]. The supine position is also a contributor to supine hypotension (low maternal blood pressure and decreased placental blood flow).

Women who are restricted to bed (e.g. for hypertension, narcotic or epidural analgesia, non-reassuring fetal heart rate responses, or institutional custom) may still be able to use position changes to improve labor progress. If the woman has back pain or other indicators of malposition, see Side-lying positions (page 116) for suggestions as to which side the mother should lie on.

If the mother does not have indicators of malposition, or if it is difficult to determine which side the fetal back is on, it is appropriate to try the 'rollover'. In the 'rollover', shown in Fig. 5.18, the bedridden woman spends 20–30 minutes in each of the following positions: semi-sitting, left side-lying, left semi-prone, hands and knees, right semi-prone, right side-lying, and back to semi-sitting . . .). She should, however, avoid any positions that she or her fetus do not tolerate well.

Unfortunately, few trials have been conducted on the effects of walking or position changes as an intervention to correct labor dystocia. The trials of ambulation in normal labor have shown no harm to women in normal labor who walk[24]. One large trial found that, when asked, 99% of the women who had been assigned to walk in labor (and did so) said they would choose to do so again[26]. Therefore, a lack of harm and high acceptance by women may be justification enough to encourage walking and position changes in labor. See

5

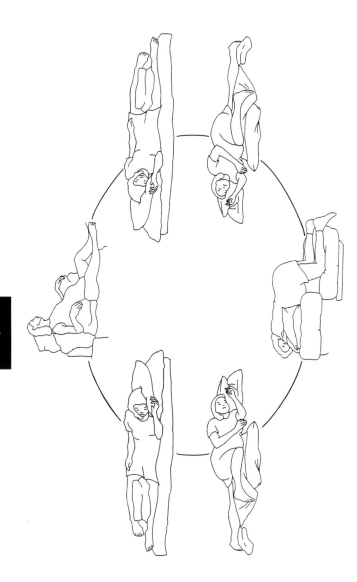

Fig. 5.18 The 'rollover sequence' for use when there are *no indicators of malposition*, or when it is *difficult to determine which side the fetal back is on*.

Chapter 7, page 235 for an explanation of how walking or stair-climbing may enhance labor progress. There may be a psychological benefit of upright positions in that a horizontal position may reinforce feelings of helplessness or powerlessness when laboring women are surrounded by people who are standing and looking down at them. By sitting or standing upright, the woman may feel more powerful and become more optimistic.

Medication

Narcotic analgesia in early labor may temporarily weaken the woman's contractions. Simply allowing medications to wear off may lead to stronger contractions, although the woman may find this intolerable.

Does the epidural interfere with labor progress? Although epidural and combined spinal epidural analgesia provide the most effective pain relief and fewest maternal mental effects, two literature reviews concluded that epidural use, compared to no epidural use, is associated with longer labors, fewer spontaneous vaginal births, more instrumental deliveries, and other undesirable side effects unrelated to labor progress[27,28]. Having an epidural on request seems to influence the rate of malpositions at delivery. A large prospective study compared outcomes of 1562 nulliparas (1437, or 92% with an epidural, 125 without)[15]. Before receiving their epidurals, the women had no greater labor pain, no more pain specifically in the back, and no more fetal malpositions than those who did not use an epidural. At delivery, however, there were 4 times more OPs in the epidural group than in the non-epidural group (12.9% vs 3.3%). The incidence of OTs was similar (8.1% vs 7.3%). The authors reported that surgical delivery rates (including instrumental deliveries and cesareans) were extremely high among women with a malpositioned fetus – 82.6% for OP and 86.5% for OT fetuses, compared to 23.8% for OA fetuses. This study indicates that elective epidurals may contribute indirectly to the cesarean and instrumental delivery rates by increasing the incidence of OP.

In the United States, epidurals are used by 80% or more of women laboring in many large urban hospitals[29], and by 63% of a combined rural and urban sample[30]. It seems clear that labor management with an epidural should include measures to enhance labor progress and facilitate fetal rotation. The Quick Epidural Index on page 290 contains references to positions and other relevant information that may contribute to lower cesarean rates for women with epidurals.

Dehydration

Most laboring women prefer to drink liquids to satisfy thirst and alleviate dryness in their mouths. If they are allowed to drink as desired and offered a beverage frequently, they will hydrate themselves adequately during labor. The 'nothing by mouth' order for healthy women in normal labor is rare, although the practice of limiting the amount and choice of fluids (e.g. sips or ice chips only, water only) is still widespread[30-32], especially with caregivers who perceive all laboring women as pre-surgical patients. These providers prefer intravenous hydration, even though it carries its own set of potential risks and drawbacks (neonatal hypoglycemia, maternal and fetal hyponatremia, maternal psychological stress, fluid overload, postpartum swelling and breast engorgement)[31]. The simplest practice to prevent dehydration is to encourage the woman to drink to thirst (water or fruit juice), and to note whether and approximately how much she is drinking.

Some women vomit frequently throughout labor, and are at higher risk of dehydration. Contrary to widely held opinion, withholding oral fluids under such circumstances does not decrease the likelihood of vomiting, though it may decrease the volume. In fact, sips of water or juice may make the woman feel better, even if she continues to vomit, but she may require intravenous fluids for adequate hydration.

Exhaustion

Fatigue or exhaustion, especially if the woman is upset or afraid, is a major concern for women experiencing long labors. Massage, music, dim light, aromatherapy, guided imagery, a bath or whatever she finds soothing may relax her and help her accept the slow pace of her labor. Reassurance from a patient and empathic caregiver can ease the woman's worry. Positions for tired women, shown in Fig. 5.19a–f, are more restful than others, and may provide a welcome change.

Note regarding food and fluids in labor

A policy of withholding food and fluids from laboring women became widespread in North America and the United Kingdom in the 1940s and 1950s and remained until the 1980s. The policy was based on concerns over the dangers of general anesthesia for laboring women who had food in their stomachs, because they were more likely to vomit and aspirate the vomitus (food particles and gastric acid) while under general anesthesia. Fasting has not been proven to solve such problems; in fact, the gastric secretions are actually more acidic and thus more damaging if aspirated than when the woman is not fasting. Safe anesthesia techniques appear to be the best safeguard against aspiration. Furthermore, the use of general anesthesia has been almost entirely replaced by epidural and spinal anesthesia (for cesareans). As a result, policies of 'nothing by mouth', at least in early labor, have declined. In fact, the risks of withholding nourishment, especially during a long labor (ketosis, hypoglycemia, maternal hunger and thirst), may be greater than the risks of general anesthesia for the low risk woman. Digestion usually slows down by active labor and the woman has little appetite for food, though she will probably want to continue to drink fluids.

Uterine lactic acidosis as a cause of inadequate contractions

5

Recent research studies indicate that in some women, occlusion of myometrial blood vessels during contractions may decrease tissue oxygen levels and cause an accumulation of lactic acid in the myometrium. This local lactic acidosis (lowered pH in myometrial capillary blood) and decreased oxygen saturation can decrease the intensity and frequency of uterine contractions[33]. In such cases augmenting with oxytocin may exacerbate the lactic acidosis, and resting the uterus (and the woman) may be more appropriate. Allowing the contractions to space out temporarily may hasten the clearance of lactic acid and the return of an efficient labor pattern. Further research on the pathophysiology, prevention, and treatment of myometrial lactic acidosis is needed to clarify the contribution of this condition to the cesarean rate. The potential benefits of identifying women with lactic acidosis during dysfunctional labor and developing methods to reverse it should be investigated.

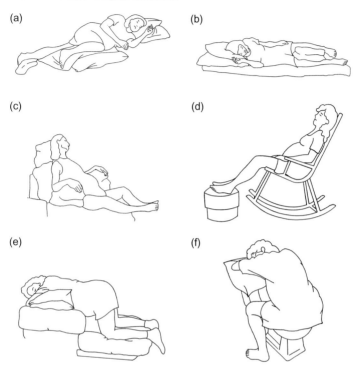

Fig. 5.19 (a) Positions for tired women: Semi-prone. (b) Side-lying. (c) Semi-sitting. (d) Sitting in a rocking chair. (e) Kneeling on foot of bed. (f) Straddling a toilet.

When the cause of inadequate contractions is unknown

Besides the techniques described in Chapter 2, 'Techniques to elicit stronger contractions', the following measures may lead to stronger contractions:

Nipple stimulation

Used for centuries to start or augment labor, nipple stimulation is frequently used by midwives and other low-intervention caregivers, especially in out-of-hospital settings. They ask the woman or her partner to lightly stroke one or both nipples to increase oxytocin release, thus augmenting contractions. When nipple stimulation is used, it is important to monitor for fetal well-being and the possibility of excessive contractions. Only one small trial has compared nipple stimulation to oxytocin for labor augmentation[34]. Because of methodological problems, reliable conclusions regarding effectiveness could not be made. The other studies of breast stimulation investigated it as a method of conducting the Contraction Stress Test, and as a method of inducing labor[35]. Case reports of nipple stimulation by high-risk women as part of a contraction stress test have described tetanic contractions. A Cochrane Review comparing breast stimulation with no treatment for labor induction found that breast stimulation increased the chances that women would go into labor within three days if they had a favorable cervix when they initiated it[35]. When compared with oxytocin, breast stimulation had similar success rates for starting labor. Uterine hyperstimulation did not occur in the low-risk women in the reviewed trials. Breast stimulation for labor augmentation, as opposed to induction, has not been studied, although it is promising as a useful technique for slow labor progress.

5

Walking and changes in position

Walking and position changes, including upright positions, improve effectiveness of contractions, and the freedom to move around improves women's satisfaction with the birth experience[24–26 and 36].

Acupressure or acupuncture

These traditional Eastern healing approaches may be used to stimulate more frequent contractions. Acupressure has never been scientifically evaluated for effectiveness or safety, although no harmful effects have been reported when it was used properly. See Chapter 8, pages 259–260, for instructions. The use of acupuncture during labor requires specialized training for the midwife or consultation with a qualified acupuncturist. While acupuncture during labor has been found to reduce pain in three trials, it has not been studied for its effectiveness in enhancing labor progress[36].

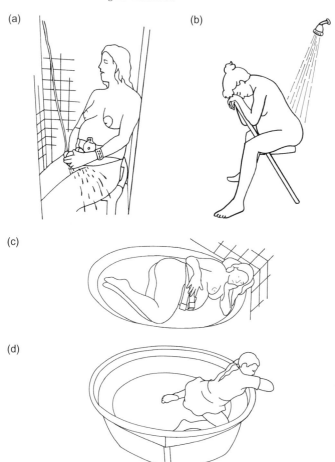

Fig. 5.20 Hydrotherapy to speed labor: (a) Shower on woman's abdomen. (b) Shower on woman's back. (c) Laboring in bath. (d) Laboring in birthing pool.

Hydrotherapy (baths and showers): Fig. 5.20a–d

Buoyancy, hydrostatic pressure, warmth, skin stimulation, and other factors induce relaxation, temporarily reduce pain awareness, and may reduce catecholamine production[37–38], and/or speed progress in active labor. Some of these benefits may be due to the relief of stress, tension, anxiety or pain. For guidelines on the use of hydrotherapy see Chapter 8, pages 252–257.

One randomized controlled trial compared usual labor augmentation procedures (amniotomy and/or oxytocin) with immersion in water for women diagnosed with dystocia. After up to four hours of immersion, the women in the bath group were reassessed for progress and, if there was not improvement in progress, they had the usual augmentation procedures. In the bath group, 29% needed no further augmentation, a significant reduction when compared to the usual care group (96% of whom received usual augmentation)[39].

Timing of the bath may be important. As stated in Chapter 4, using the bath in early labor may slow the contractions, whereas using it in the active phase often speeds dilation[39].

In summary, contractions may be slowed or weakened by policies that restrict movement, withhold food or drink, raise maternal anxiety, overmedicate the woman, or medicate her too early in labor. A policy of prevention by avoiding such policies seems desirable, since the effects are difficult to reverse with physiological interventions. If the above measures fail to improve the effectiveness of contractions, then artificial rupture of the membranes and/or intravenous oxytocin may become necessary.

IF THERE IS A PERSISTENT CERVICAL LIP OR A SWOLLEN CERVIX

Position changes can often be used to reduce a persistent cervical lip (that is, a cervix that is fully dilated except for an anterior lip) or to reduce a swollen cervix, which may become increasingly edematous without treatment. A cervical lip is thought to be formed either by uneven pressure by the presenting part on the cervix or by the anterior cervix becoming caught between the fetal head and pubic arch. The following approaches may correct the problem.

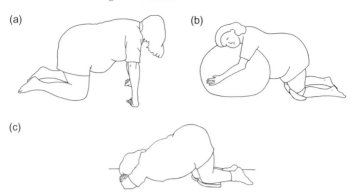

Fig. 5.21 (a) Hands and knees. (b) Kneeling with a ball and knee pads. (c) Open knee–chest position.

Position changes to reduce an anterior lip or a swollen cervix

Often the woman seems to know what to do. When free to seek more comfortable positions she is likely to choose a position that helps reduce the anterior lip or swelling. If that does not succeed, time and positions that reduce the pressure of the fetal head or pubic arch on the cervix seem to be the best positions to use. Gravity-neutral or anti-gravity positions, such as hands and knees, kneeling with a ball or the open knee–chest position (Fig. 5.21a–c) may move the fetal head away from the cervix and take some of the pressure off. Side-lying, semi-prone, or standing positions (Fig. 5.22a–d) redistribute the pressure on the cervix and may reduce a lip.

Other methods

Immersion in deep water: the 'weightlessness' and buoyancy reduce the effects of gravity and may relieve pressure on the cervix. We are intrigued by a suggestion in a midwifery text for reducing swelling in the cervix, by filling the finger of a sterile glove with crushed ice and applying it to the cervix[41]. We have no experience with this and there are no published studies of this technique.

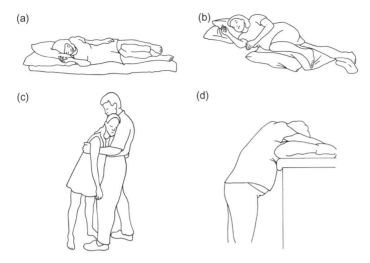

Fig. 5.22 (a) Side-lying. (b) Semi-prone, lower arm forward. (c) Standing, leaning on partner. (d) Standing, leaning on counter.

Note on asynclitism and the occiput posterior (OP) position:

Asymmetrical dilation (and the formation of a cervical lip) often occurs when the fetus is asynclitic or OP. See pages 112–120, for positions that may resolve these malpositions.

MANUAL REDUCTION OF A PERSISTENT CERVICAL LIP

Sometimes, if patience, position changes, or the bath do not succeed in reducing the lip, manual reduction may be warranted[13]. The technique, used by many midwives, nurses, and physicians, is explained below:

- Explain the procedure, along with the expected benefit of shortening the time until complete dilation. Tell her that it will be painful, and gain the mother's consent and cooperation.
- Begin by placing two fingers between the head and the lip of cervix before the onset of a contraction.

- Instruct the mother (who may or may not be experiencing a spontaneous urge to push) *not* to push until you tell her to do so.
- As you feel the contraction begin, push the cervix behind the head. If it moves easily, instruct the mother to push, to help the head advance, leaving the lip behind it.
- Check after the contraction to be sure that the lip has not reappeared.
- Repeat if necessary and if the mother can tolerate it.

IF EMOTIONAL DYSTOCIA IS SUSPECTED

The term 'emotional dystocia' refers to dysfunctional labor caused by emotional distress and the resulting excessive production of catecholamines. High catecholamine levels can reduce the circulation to the uterus and placenta during labor, causing inefficient contractions and reduced fetal oxygenation. In addition, according to Michel Odent[42], constant disturbance in a busy, strange environment may make it difficult or impossible for the woman to relax mentally or physically, 'turn off' her neo-cortex, and labor instinctually, as explained in Chapter 2. Chapter 2 also explains the psychobiological basis of emotional dystocia.

Assessing the woman's coping

Western cultural attitudes on coping with labor

Childbirth education programs first emerged in the 1940s, when much less was known about the powerful, multisensory ways in which women spontaneously cope with labor. Much has been learned since then, but older ideas have left their stamp on Western culture, and seem to be reiterated endlessly by popular media. Many people still think that 'coping well' means that the woman remains silent and does not move during contractions. Often, caregivers, partners, and the women themselves believe that women who are physically active and vocal are coping poorly, and may strive to help these women to be quiet. However, we now know that women with kinesthetic and vocal coping styles often find much more effective relief from pain and stress when they move and make sounds, than when they try to use the quiet, still techniques of the early childbirth methods.

The essence of 'coping' during the first stage of labor

When we look closely at active vocal women, we notice that some follow a rhythm and others vocalize irregularly and move jerkily, without rhythm. The women whose activities are rhythmic and repetitious are actually coping well, even though they may be loud and active.

Rhythm is the common element in coping during the first stage of labor, just as it is the key to success in physical endurance events, and some kinds of meditation, yoga, and self-calming techniques. Rhythmic breathing, vocalizing, swaying, tapping, self-stroking, even rhythmic mental activities, such as counting breaths through a contraction, repeating a mantra or verse, or singing a song aloud or to herself, are all examples of ways women use rhythm as a coping technique. Usually, by the time a woman is in active labor, she is no longer using techniques she was taught in prenatal classes, although these may have been helpful earlier. Rhythmic activities in active labor are unique and unplanned. They emerge spontaneously when women are not afraid and are not disturbed or restricted in their behavior. When women begin to develop these spontaneous rhythmic behaviors, the cognitive parts of their brains are less active and their behavior becomes more instinctual. In fact, women often express surprise later at the repetitive rhythmic behaviors they discovered during labor, and how effective they were.

Other spontaneous coping behaviors exhibited by these women include relaxation during and/or between contractions, and routines, or 'rituals', which are the repetition of the same rhythmic activities for many contractions in a row. Coping rituals often involve other people (the partner, doula, or someone else) and the mother wants them to continue doing the same comforting behaviors with each contraction. They may hold her, stroke or sway with her, speak to her or moan softly in her rhythm, and help her regain her rhythm if she loses it. These three: relaxation, rhythm, and ritual, are referred to as the 3 Rs. They constitute the essence of coping during the first stage of labor.

The caregiver, in assessing the woman's well-being during labor, should observe her coping behavior. If she has rhythm in whatever she is doing, she is coping; if she has lost her rhythm, she needs help to regain it. See also page 142, 'if the source of the woman's anxiety cannot be identified,' for more on assessing the woman's emotional state.

In summary, 'coping well' during labor and birth often includes instinctive vocalization, movement, and self-comforting behavior. During the first stage, relaxation, rhythm and ritual are good signs of coping.

Indicators of emotional dystocia during active labor

A woman experiencing emotional dystocia may do some of the following:

- Express or display fear or anxiety
- Lack rhythm and ritual in her responses to contractions
- Ask many questions, or remain very alert to her surroundings
- Exhibit very 'needy' behavior
- Display extreme modesty
- Exhibit strong reactions to mild contractions or to examinations
- Show a high degree of muscle tension
- Appear demanding, distrustful, angry, or resentful toward staff
- Seem hypervigilant, highly alert, 'jumpy', or easily startled
- Exhibit a strong need for control over caregivers' actions
- Seem 'out of control' in labor (in extreme pain, writhing, pan-icked, screaming, unresponsive to helpful suggestions or questions)
- Express fear that she will lose control as labor becomes more intense
- Or she may not exhibit any external behaviors that would lead one to consider emotional dystocia. (See pages 92–93, pages 137–138 and pages 265–266, for ways to discover whether fear or anxiety may be contributing to the dystocia.)

Predisposing factors for emotional dystocia

Whatever the woman's fears or anxieties are, she probably cannot simply 'snap out of it'. Her emotional state results partly from pre-existing factors, which may include:

- Previous difficult births
- Previous traumatic hospitalizations
- Childhood abuse: physical, sexual, or emotional (see pages 139–141 on the impact of sexual abuse on childbearing women)
- Dysfunctional family of origin (mental illness, substance abuse, fighting by parents, or other family problems)

- Fears about current serious health problems
- Domestic violence (previous or present)
- Cultural factors, including beliefs leading to extreme shame when viewed nude, or when viewed in labor by men or when behaving in a way that is contrary to cultural expectations
- Language barriers, or inability to hear or understand what is happening or being done
- Substance abuse by the woman
- Death of her own mother (especially in childbirth or at a young age)
- Beliefs resulting from what she has been told about labor (e.g. the woman whose sibling was handicapped by a 'birth injury', or whose mother had a 'terrible time' giving birth to her)

Helping the woman state her fears

Of course, maternity professionals are not expected to provide psychotherapy. On the other hand, addressing her concerns by asking a few sensitive questions between contractions may help the woman state her fears and allow those around her to give more effective care: 'What was going through your mind during that contraction?' or 'How are you feeling right now?', or 'Do you have any idea why your labor is slowing down?' She may indicate any of the following common fears or others, which could interfere with labor progress:

- Dread of increasing pain
- Fear of damage or disfigurement to her own body, including stretching, episiotomy, tears, stitching, or a cesarean, and 'never being the same again'
- Fear of uterine rupture, if she has had a cesarean before
- Fear that labor will harm her baby (a belief that a cesarean is safer and easier for the baby)
- Fear of loss of control, of modesty, or of dignity; 'acting like a fool' or 'losing face' (shame)
- Fear of invasive procedures, such as vaginal exams, injections, blood tests or others
- Fear of her caregivers, many or all of whom may be unknown to her (she may perceive them as strangers who have power and authority over her)

- Fear of being unable to care for her baby adequately, of being a 'terrible mother'
- Fear of abandonment by the baby's father, her caregiver, or others
- Fear of dying (Note: a brief transient period of fear of dying in the late first stage, associated with a surge of catecholamines and the 'fetal ejection reflex' (see pages 17–18) is not unusual, and it is not associated with dystocia[43]. A deep, prolonged, persistent fear throughout pregnancy and labor is what we are referring to here.)

It is important to acknowledge that most women have some fear or anxiety about labor, birth, and the impact of a new child on their lives. This does not mean that all those women will have labor dystocia. For some women, however, emotional issues are powerful enough to interfere with an efficient labor pattern. Being able to recognize and help those women may reduce the negative impact of emotional distress. In any case, your sensitivity and attentiveness will contribute to a woman's sense of being cared for and cared about.

How to help a laboring woman in distress

After having identified (or, having guessed) the woman's fears, it may be helpful to do some or all of the following:

- Provide language interpreters and culturally competent or culturally sensitive caregivers, if needed.

- Restate what she has said to check that you understand ('It sounds as if you're afraid of what the labor might do to your baby. Is that right?'). If the woman confirms this, then:

- Validate her fear, rather than dismissing it. 'Yes, other women have told me they worried about that too,' or 'That must be frightening. We're also concerned about babies during labor and that's why we check your baby's heartbeat frequently.'

- Provide reassuring information (but not empty promises). 'As I listen to his heartbeat, he sounds just fine right now. Would you like to know how babies adapt to contractions during labor? They have some really amazing coping mechanisms . . .'

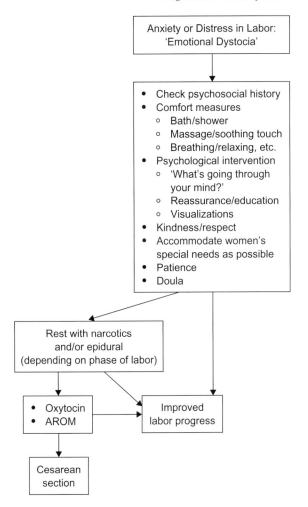

Chart 5.4 Anxiety or distress in labor.

- Observe her face and behavior during conversations and elicit further concerns or needs.

- Between contractions let her know that, after the baby is born, there are helpful resources available to her (and follow up with this information later). For example, if the woman is worried about being an inadequate mother, she might be relieved to know there are parenting classes and support groups, and a hotline she can call for help at any time, day or night. Helping her recognize that labor is not the time to address her fears about parenthood, while also reassuring her that she will not be alone with her concerns, may ease her anxiety enough that labor progress will resume. Perhaps calming her conscious fears will help her enter a more relaxed state in which the 'primitive' parts of her brain will predominate and promote the labor process.

- Provide ideas (non-judgmentally) that the woman can use to alter the situation. If the woman feels 'helpless' lying down, she might feel strong and active standing up.

- Visualization and reframing can be powerful tools to help a woman overcome her fear. For example, if she expresses concern about her 'poor baby's head being forced through that tiny tight opening', she can be helped to imagine her 'little baby nuzzling his head down in that soft stretchy place' (describing her ripe cervix and vagina as being as soft and stretchy as the inside of her cheek when she presses inside it with her tongue).

- If the woman is unable to cope with overwhelming physical sensations, she may benefit from massage, hydrotherapy, or pain medication.

Chart 5.4 summarizes ways to help women when emotional distress is a likely cause of dystocia. See below for a summary of the special needs of childhood abuse survivors.

Special needs of childhood abuse survivors[44]

A woman who was sexually or physically abused as a child may have great anxieties in labor, especially related to:

- Invasive procedures that remind her of the abuse, such as: vaginal exams, instruments placed in the vagina, blood draws, or IVs.
- Lack of control: as a child she was hurt when she was out of control and vulnerable. She may have learned never to lose control.
- Modesty, nakedness, exposure issues.
- Powerful authority figures (midwives, nurses, doctors) who know more than she, and who do painful things to her: as a child she was a victim of those with authority over her.
- Being asked to 'relax, surrender, or yield to the contractions' with the promise that it won't hurt so much: she may have been told similar things during the abuse.
- Pushing her baby out of her vagina: the pain and prospect of damage may remind her of sexual abuse.

Sometimes an abuse survivor responds emotionally or angrily in the above situations. The caregiver should not take her reaction personally and should keep in mind that the woman has very good reason to react the way she does, and also that the caregiver is not the reason. If a caregiver observes some of the behaviors listed above, she or he should suspect a history of sexual or another type of abuse, and try to be patient and kind, listen to her, and meet her special needs to the extent possible, even if they seem unusual or unreasonable. If she feels emotionally safe, her labor may progress more normally, and she may reap other psychological benefits as well.

Incompatibility or poor relationship with staff

If the woman has developed a poor relationship with any staff member, it will help to have a discussion with the staff member or with that person's superior regarding the specific concerns or differences of opinion. Sometimes all the woman needs is to be listened to, respected, and taken seriously, so that she may be more able to trust the people around her. Perhaps the staff will be able to make some compromises in their usual routines in order to meet her needs, while still accomplishing those clinical tasks that are essential to basic safety.

The simplest solution, once the woman discovers that she and her nurse or midwife are incompatible, is to change to someone else to provide a fresh start in the relationship. There is no need to lay blame, only to recognize the incompatibility and correct it.

If it is possible to anticipate these difficulties before labor, it makes sense to suggest that this patient be assigned to a particularly diplomatic or understanding midwife or nurse, and that the woman brings a doula (professional labor support person) with her in labor. The doula can provide extra psychological support to relieve the burden on the caregiver.

If the source of the woman's anxiety cannot be identified

Sometimes a caregiver cannot understand why the labor is not going well. All the physical factors seem normal, and the woman does not exhibit any particular psychosocial problems. It sometimes helps to wait until after a contraction and ask her, 'Could you tell me what was going through your mind during that contraction?' If necessary, ask, 'Anything else?' The answer she gives may be a clue to her emotional state. For example, if she responds, 'I am just trying to do the breathing and relaxation I learned in childbirth class,' it is clear that she is coping, and should be encouraged to continue the self-comforting measures. If, however, she says she is afraid, or feels helpless, or it hurts terribly, or she cannot do it for much longer, she is obviously in distress, and needs more emotional support. The caregiver can help (in culturally appropriate ways) by acknowledging her distress, reassuring her, addressing her fear, holding her hand, and helping her and her partner with some self-comforting measures. (See Chapter 2.) One notable study found that women who expressed distress in early labor were more likely to have longer labors, more fetal distress, and all the interventions that go along with these problems[45]. If emotional distress can be identified and alleviated early in labor with extra support, reassurance, encouragement, and assistance, these damaging effects of distress may be prevented.

In summary, the psycho-emotional factors that influence labor progress are less well understood than the physical factors, but they may be as important. Try to remain sensitive to this aspect of childbirth. Your influence on the mind–body connection in labor may be greater than you think.

CONCLUSION

Labor progress may slow in active labor for a variety of reasons. We have provided guidelines for determining the possible cause. When mother and fetus are faring well, interventions or actions specific to the cause may be used to address the problem. Sometimes more than one cause exists for a problem, and several measures are appropriate.

REFERENCES

1. O'Driscoll, K., Meagher, D. & Boylan, P. (1993) *Active Management of Labour*. Mosby Year Book Europe, London.
2. Friedman, E.A. (1995) Dystocia and 'failure to progress' in labor. In: *Cesarean Section: Guidelines for Appropriate Utilization* (eds B.L. Flamm & E.J. Quilligan). Springer-Verlag, New York.
3. Sweet, B. & Tiran, D. (eds) (1997) *Mayes' Midwifery: a Textbook for Midwives*, 12th edn. Baillière Tindall, London.
4. Enkin, M., Keirse, M., Neilsen, J., *et al.* (2000) Monitoring the progress of labour. In: *A Guide to Effective Care in Pregnancy and Childbirth*, 3rd edn. Oxford University Press, Oxford.
5. Zhang, J., Troendle, J. & Yancey, M. (2002) Reassessing the labor curve in nulliparous women. *American Journal of Obstetrics and Gynecology*, **187**, 824–8.
6. Page, L.A. (ed.) (2000) *The New Midwifery: Science and Sensitivity in Practice*. Churchill Livingstone, Edinburgh.
7. Sinclair, C. (2004) *A Midwife's Handbook*. Saunders, St Louis.
8. Sutton, J. (2001) *Let Birth Be Born Again: Rediscovering and Reclaiming Our Midwifery Heritage*. Birth Concepts, Bedfont, Middlesex, UK.
9. King, J.M. (1993) *Back Labor No More!! What Every Woman Should Know Before Labor*. Plenary Systems, Dallas.
10. Fitzpatrick, M., McQuillan, K. & O'Herlihy, C. (2001) Influence of persistent occiput posterior position of delivery outcome. *Obstetrics and Gynecology*, **98**, 1027–31.
11. Gardberg, M., Laakonen E. & Salevaara, M. (1998) Intrapartum sonography and persistent occiput posterior position: a study of 408 deliveries. *Obstetrics and Gynecology*, **91**, 746–9.
12. Ponkey, S., Cohen, A., Heffner, L. & Lieberman, E. (2003) Persistent fetal occiput posterior position: obstetric outcomes. *Obstetrics and Gynecology*, **101**(5.1), 915–20.
13. Varney, H. (2003) *Varney's Midwifery*, 4th edn. Jones & Bartlett, Boston.
14. Hofmeyr, G. (2004) Obstructed labor: using better technologies to reduce mortality. *International Journal of Gynecology and Obstetrics*, **85**, Suppl.1; S62–S72.
15. Lieberman, E., Davidson, K., Lee-Parritz, A., Shearer, E. (2005) Changes in fetal position during labor and their association with epidural analgesia. *Obstetrics and Gynecology*, 105, 974–82.

5

16. Fraser, W., Vendittelli, F., Krauss, I. & Breart, G. (1998) Effects of early augmentation of labour with amniotomy and oxytocin in nulliparous women: a meta-analysis. *British Journal of Obstetrics and Gynaecology*, **105**, 189–94.

17. ACOG (2003) Clinical management Guidelines for Obstetrician–Gynecologists. *Dystocia and Augmentation of Labor*. ACOG Practice Bulletin no. 49. American College of Obstetricians and Gynecologists, Washington, DC.

18. Schwarcz, R., Diaz, A., Belizan, J., Fescina, R. & Caldeyro-Barcia, R. (1976) Proceedings of the VIII World Congress of Gynecology and Obstetrics. Excerpta Medica Amsterdam, Mexico City.

19. Michel, S., Rake, A., Treiber, K., *et al.* (2002) MR obstetric pelvimetry: effect of birthing position on pelvic bony dimensions. *American Journal of Roentgenology*, **179**, 1063–67.

20. Simkin, P. (2003) Maternal positions and pelves revisited. *Birth*, **30**, 130–32.

21. Scott, P. (2003) *Sit Up and Take Notice! Positioning Yourself for a Better Birth*. Great Scott Publications, New Zealand.

22. Andrews, C. & Andrews, E. (1983) Nursing, maternal postures, and fetal position. *Nursing Research*, **32**, 336–41.

23. Fenwick, L. & Simkin, P. (1987) Maternal positioning to prevent or alleviate dystocia. *Clinical Obstetrics and Gynecology*, **30**(1), 83–9.

24. Roberts, J. (1989) Maternal position during the first stage of labour. In: *Effective Care in Pregnancy and Childbirth*, vol. 2, (eds I. Chalmers, M. Enkin & M. Keirse). Oxford University Press, Oxford.

25. Simkin, P. & O'Hara. (2002) Nonpharmacologic relief of pain during labor: systematic reviews of five methods. *American Journal of Obstetrics and Gynecology*, **186**, S131–S159.

26. Bloom, S.L., McIntire, D.D., Kelly, M.A., *et al.* (1998) Lack of effect of walking on labor and delivery. *New England Journal of Medicine*, **339**, 76–9.

27. Lieberman, E. & O'Donoghue, C. (2002) Unintended effects of epidural analgesia during labor: a systematic review. *American Journal of Obstetrics & Gynecology*, **186**, S31–S68.

28. Leighton, B. (2002) The effects of epidural analgesia on labor, maternal, and neonatal outcomes: a systematic review. *American Journal of Obstetrics & Gynecology*, **186**, S69–S77.

29. Great Starts Birth & Family Education (2004) *Great Starts' Birth Services Survey: Regional Hospitals, Midwifery Services, and Out-of Hospital Birth Services*. Great Starts, Seattle.

30. DeClerq, E., Sakala, C., Corry, M., Applebaum, S. & Risher, P. (2002) *Listening to Mothers: Report of the First National US Survey of Women's Childbearing Experiences*. Maternity Center Association/Harris Interactive, New York.

31. Kroeger, M. & Smith, L. (2004) *Impact of Birthing Practices on Breast-feeding: Protecting the Mother and Baby Continuum.* Jones & Bartlett, Boston.

32. Enkin, M., Keirse, M., Neilsen, J., *et al.* (2000) *A Guide to Effective Care in Pregnancy and Childbirth*, 3rd edn. Oxford University Press, Oxford.

33. Quenby, S., Pierce, S., Brigham, S. & Wray, S. (2004) Dysfunctional labor and myometrial lactic acidosis. *Obstetrics and Gynecology*, **103**, 718–23.

34. Curtis, P., Resnick, J., Evens, S. & Thompson, C. (1999) A comparison of breast stimulation and intravenous oxytocin for the augmentation of labor. *Birth*, **29**, 115–22.

35. Kavanaugh, J., Kelly, A. & Thomas, J. (2001) Breast stimulation for cervical ripening and induction of labour. The Cochrane Database of Systematic Reviews 2001, Issue 4. Art. No.: CD003392. DOI:10.1002/14651858.CD003392.

36. Simkin, P. & Bolding, A. (2004) Update on non-pharmacological approaches to relieve labor pain and prevent suffering. *Journal of Midwifery and Womens Health*, **49**, 489–504.

37. Odent, M. (1997) Can water immersion stop labor? *Journal of Nurse-Midwifery*, **42**, 414–16.

38. Grossman, E., Goldstein, D., Hoffman, S., Wacks, I. & Epstein, M. (1992) Effects of water immersion on sympathoadrenal and dopamine systems in humans. *American Journal of Physiology*, **262**, R993–9.

39. Cluett, E., Pickering, R., Getliffe, K. & Saunders, N. (2004) Random-ized controlled trial of labouring in water compared with standard of augmentation of dystocia in first stage of labour. *British Medical Journal*, doi:10.1136/bmj.37963.606412.EE: 1–6.

40. Eriksson, M., Mattson, L.A. & Ladfors, L. (1997) Early or late bath during the first stage of labour: a randomised study of 200 women. *Midwifery*, **13**, 146–8.

41. Davis, E. (1997) *Heart and Hands: A Midwife's Guide to Pregnancy and Birth*, 3rd edn. Celestial Arts, Berkeley.

42. Odent, M. (1999) Birth reborn, Chapter 6. In: *The Scientification of Love.* Free Association Books, London.

43. Odent, M. (1992) *The Nature of Birth and Breastfeeding.* Bergin & Garvey, Westport, Conn.

44. Simkin, P. & Klaus, P. (2004) *When Survivors Give Birth: Understanding and Healing the Effects of Early Sexual Abuse on Childbearing Women.* Classic Day Publishing, Seattle.

45. Wuitchik, M., Bakal, D. & Lipshitz, J. (1989) The clinical significance of pain and cognitive activity in latent labor. *Obstetrics and Gynecology*, **73**(1), 35–41.

5

Chapter 6

Prolonged Second Stage of Labor

Definitions of the second stage of labor, 146
The phases of the second stage, 147
The latent phase of the second stage, 147
The active phase of the second stage, 150
If the woman has an epidural, 156
How long an active phase of second stage is too long? 161
Possible etiologies and solutions for second-stage dystocia, 162
Positions and other strategies for suspected occiput posterior (OP) or
    persistent occiput transverse (OT) fetuses, 162
Why not the dorsal position? 162
Differentiating between pushing positions and birth positions, 165
Manual interventions to reposition the OP fetus, 174
Early interventions for suspected persistent asynclitism, 174
If cephalo-pelvic disproportion (CPD) or macrosomia is suspected, 177
Positions for 'possible CPD' in second stage, 178
Shoulder dystocia, 188
If contractions are inadequate, 188
If emotional dystocia is suspected, 188
Conclusion, 192
References, 193

DEFINITIONS OF THE SECOND STAGE OF LABOR

By definition, the second stage of labor begins with complete dilation of the cervix and ends with the birth of the baby. The clinical significance of complete dilation is controversial. There are two basic schools of thought regarding the conduct of the second stage. One is based on a desire for a speedy delivery, and calls for the woman to commence maximal breath-holding and bearing-down (pushing) efforts when she is discovered to be fully dilated, even though her urge to push may occur before or after complete dilation. If the urge to push occurs before complete dilation, the woman is told to resist pushing by panting throughout each contraction (see pages 120–122 for further discussion of what to do with a premature urge to push). If the urge to push is not present when she is completely dilated, the desire for a speedy delivery leads the caregiver to exhort the woman to begin pushing.

This approach has begun to give way to a less hurried approach, in which being completely dilated, in itself, is not believed to be sufficient reason to begin pushing. Rather, the conduct of second stage is based on complete dilation plus involuntary expulsive efforts (an urge to push). This approach has a basis in physiology since, in the normal course of events, contractions sometimes diminish temporarily around the time of full dilation. With this less hurried approach, the woman begins pushing later and pushes less than with the former approach.

THE PHASES OF THE SECOND STAGE

The second stage of labor can be divided into phases (the latent phase and the active phase), just as the first stage is. Each phase represents different maternal behaviors and different physiological accomplishments.

The latent phase of the second stage

6

An apparent lull in uterine activity around the time of complete dilation is frequently observed and is sometimes referred to as the 'latent phase of the second stage'[1], the 'resting phase'[2], or the 'rest and be thankful phase'[3]. There are no reports of the frequency with which a noticeable lull actually occurs, although it is a phenomenon widely recognized by maternity professionals. How and why it occurs is not fully understood, but there are interesting hypotheses.

Let us review what happens to the uterus during the first stage of labor (Fig. 6.1). During most of the first stage, the uterus is tightly wrapped around the fetus. Uterine contractions in the first stage not only dilate the cervix, but also shorten the uterine muscle fibers, and these actions gradually reduce the intrauterine space and press the fetus down.

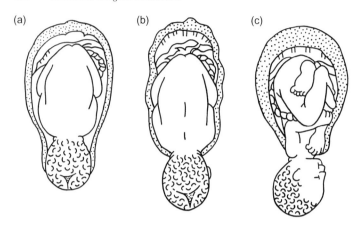

Fig. 6.1 a, b and c Latent phase of second stage. Fetal head slips through cervix, and uterine muscle slackens. Uterine muscle fibers shorten until the uterus is once again tightly wrapped around fetal trunk. (a) Fetus in uterus at full dilation. (b) Head out of uterus, which slackens. (c) Uterus shortened and thickened around fetal torso.

The last 2 cm of dilation are accompanied by cervical retraction around the head (or presenting part), and the beginnings of descent of the head into the vaginal canal[4,5]. The fetal head represents 25–30% of its entire body. Simkin's hypothesis suggests that when the head (representing a quarter of the contents of the uterus) slips through the cervix, the uterine muscle slackens as it is no longer tightly stretched around the entire fetus, and the uterus must now shrink to 'catch up' with the fetus[1].

This 'catching up' consists of shortening of the uterine muscle fibers (as happened gradually in the first stage), further reducing the intrauterine space until, once again, the uterine muscle is tightly wrapped around the fetal trunk. This may take minutes or longer, during which the woman's contractions are weak or unnoticeable, and the woman may doze. The contractions resume and the woman experiences an increasingly powerful urge to push, accompanied by a documented spurt in oxytocin release[6–8]. Only some women, however, experience such a lull. Fetal position and station may be two of the factors that determine whether and when the woman will experience a resting phase, and also how long it lasts.

This hypothesis is consistent with our knowledge of uterine physiology in labor, with Friedman's classic observations of normal labor progress, and with the numerous observational studies of maternal spontaneous bearing-down efforts that document an increasing urge to push and greater spontaneous bearing-down efforts with time and descent of the presenting part[9–10].

A second hypothesis to explain the rest early in the second stage is offered by Roberts as follows[11]. During the latent phase, contractions continue, and are measurable by electronic monitoring, although they may be below the threshold of the woman's awareness. These cause fetal rotation, alignment and descent. Women exhibit less pain and distress than earlier in labor because of the retraction of the cervix around the descending fetal head, as described by Friedman[4–5]. Women begin to experience involuntary bearing-down efforts once the fetal head is at a + 1 station and has rotated to occiput anterior, and the contractions have achieved and maintained an intensity of 30 mm Hg.

Asking women to push during the latent phase of the second stage

During the latent phase, in which the uterine activity is markedly reduced, the fetal heart tones usually remain reassuring. With no interventions at all, powerful pushing contractions usually resume within 5–30 minutes. During the latent phase, the woman gets some rest, her spirits rise, and she begins to look forward to delivering her child.

Caregivers who subscribe to the approach of speeding the delivery sometimes misinterpret the latent phase to mean labor has slowed down, and make efforts to speed the second stage, by enlisting the woman's maximal bearing-down efforts, which are exhausting and non-productive because of the absence of adequate contractions or an urge to push, or by ordering intravenous oxytocin to augment uterine contractions. Though widely used to augment labor, oxytocin is not free from potential adverse effects, such as tetanic contractions and fetal distress[12].

These unnecessary interventions are less likely to be used by those who recognize the existence of distinct phases of the second stage. 'In uncomplicated labour, the timing of the decision to encourage maternal effort is usually when the presenting part is "on view" or there is obvious descent of the presenting part with an uncontrollable urge to push'[13-14].

What if the latent phase of the second stage persists?

If the lull in uterine activity persists for more than 20 or 30 minutes, the caregiver may continue monitoring and waiting, or may initiate measures to bring on contractions and an urge to push. These measures may include a change in the woman's position to sitting upright (in bed or on the toilet), squatting, or walking; 'trial' expulsive efforts (breath-holding and bearing down) by the woman; acupressure; and nipple stimulation. See the Toolkit in Chapter 8 and pages 32, 129 for specific descriptions and precautions regarding these measures.

Many professionals now await evidence of an urge to push before checking the woman's cervix. By doing so, they are less likely to perceive second stage as prolonged. They prefer the two-fold definition of second stage: complete dilation plus spontaneous expulsive efforts.

The active phase of the second stage

The active phase of the second stage is characterized by an involuntary urge to push and descent of the fetus. It is sometimes referred to as the 'pelvic division' of labor[3], the 'press period'[11], or the descent phase[1]. The woman's contractions, her expulsive efforts, her body positions and fetal efforts are the forces that combine to bring about the delivery. Recent research regarding expulsive efforts (positions, breathing, bearing down) for second stage has resulted in some new thinking about how women should push, and the role of clinical personnel in assisting the woman at this time.

Directed expulsive efforts

Just how a woman should 'push' is the subject of some disagreement among caregivers. According to one school of thought the woman should remain horizontal, flat on her back, in a semi-reclining position or on her side. When the contraction begins, she is to draw her legs up and curl her body, take a deep breath, hold it, and strain (bear down) maximally for at least 10 seconds. Then she is to release her breath; quickly take another; and repeat this routine until the contraction ends. The caregiver actively, enthusiastically, and sometimes loudly directs these efforts.

This technique of maximal maternal effort was devised by natural childbirth advocates in the 1950s as a way to overcome the antigravity effects of the mandatory lithotomy position, and to deliver the baby quickly enough to avoid forceps[15]. It was incorporated into obstetric, nursing, and midwifery practices and continues to be a widespread practice today. There are problems with this approach, however.

Physiological effects of prolonged breath-holding and straining on the woman

Prolonged breath-holding and straining lead to:

- A closed pressure system in her chest, which leads to decreases in venous return, cardiac output, and maternal arterial blood pressure.
- An increase in the peripheral stasis of blood in her head, face, arms, and legs. Her face reddens and if an intravenous line is in place, blood often backs up in the IV catheter.
- A decrease in maternal blood oxygen levels and blood flow to the placenta.
- An increase in maternal carbon dioxide levels until she gasps for air.
- A sudden increase in her blood pressure as she gasps for air, causing bursting of tiny blood vessels in the whites of her eyes, her face, neck, and eyes (petechial hemorrhages).
- Rapid distension of the vaginal canal and pelvic musculature, along with stretching of supportive ligaments, leading to perineal trauma and possible urinary stress incontinence.
- Maternal exhaustion.

These effects are well tolerated by young healthy women, but may present risks for older or high-risk women and those with residual pelvic floor weakness, especially if such efforts are required for several hours.

MATERNAL EFFECTS:

Prolonged breath-holding and straining (Valsalva maneuver)

$\rightarrow$ a closed pressure system in chest, $\rightarrow$ $\downarrow$ venous return, $\downarrow$ cardiac output, $\downarrow$ blood pressure, and $\downarrow$ blood flow to placenta.

Also $\uparrow$ in peripheral stasis of blood (head and face, arms and legs) $\rightarrow$ red face.

Mother's O_2 levels $\downarrow$, and CO_2 levels $\uparrow$, $\rightarrow$ gasping for air, $\rightarrow$ sudden $\uparrow$ in blood pressure, $\rightarrow$ bursting of capillaries in face, neck, and eyes (petechial hemorrhages).

FETAL EFFECTS:

$\downarrow$ O_2 content in maternal arterial blood and $\downarrow$ blood flow to placenta $\rightarrow$ $\downarrow$ O_2 available to fetus (fetal hypoxia).

Chart 6.1   The prolonged Valsalva maneuver (breath-holding and straining).

Physiological effects of prolonged breath-holding and straining on the fetus

Fetal bradycardias sometimes occur when the woman holds her breath for prolonged periods and her straining may increase fetal head compression. If such bearing-down efforts are combined with a dorsal position, supine hypotension may exacerbate the bradycardia.

The decreases in maternal blood pressure, blood oxygen content, and placental blood flow cause a decrease in the oxygen available to the fetus (fetal hypoxia and acidosis)[14]. See Chart 6.1 for a summary of these effects of prolonged breath-holding and straining. These effects are well tolerated by a healthy, well nourished, term fetus, but may distress the fetus who is pre-term, small for gestational age, already compromised earlier in labor, or is experiencing cord compression.

Furthermore, such a bearing-down technique, while it may slightly shorten the second stage when compared with spontaneous bearing-down efforts, is not associated with better neonatal outcomes[10 and 16]. Perineal damage is increased (denervation, muscle damage, later incontinence) when women bear down forcefully in unfavorable positions[11 and 17].

Spontaneous expulsive efforts

Observational studies of women's behavior in the second stage reveal that women who are not directed in pushing breathe more and bear down less during second stage contractions than women who are directed to use prolonged maximal bearing-down efforts[9–10]. Also, undirected women change positions more[10 and 18]. With spontaneous bearing down in various positions, the undesirable side effects of both prolonged maximal breath-holding and the supine position do not occur.

If a woman is not required to push in a prescribed manner or in a prescribed position, she may use a number of positions (side-lying, semi-reclining, standing, a supported squat, hands and knees, kneeling on one or both knees, or squatting). She may hold her breath, moan, or even bellow during the contractions[19].

Most women experience an involuntary urge to push that comes and goes several times during each contraction. The woman's spontaneous bearing-down efforts last approximately 5–7 seconds, and she takes several breaths between bearing-down efforts[1,9,10,11,13,20]. As the second stage progresses and the fetus descends, the woman's spontaneous bearing-down efforts usually become more forceful and more frequent[9].

The caregiver's role is different when the woman is pushing spontaneously in physiological positions from when she is expected to push maximally in a supine position. In the former, the caregiver encourages and praises the woman's efforts and reassures her that her sensations are normal. The caregiver emphasizes the value of relaxing her perineum rather than holding her breath or pushing to a count of ten. Chart 6.2 illustrates the caregiver's step-by-step approach to bearing-down (pushing) efforts once dilation is complete.

Diffuse pushing

Sometimes the woman's spontaneous pushing is unfocused, or 'diffuse', and may result in little progress (Chart 6.3). It is almost as if all her effort has no single direction. Such diffuse pushing seems to occur when the woman's eyes are tightly closed, and there may be little or no apparent progress after 20 or 30 minutes. If she is making progress with diffuse pushing, there is no reason to intervene,

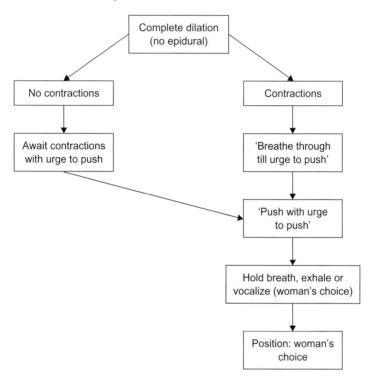

Chart 6.2   Spontaneous bearing down.

6

unless she seems distressed. If she is not making progress the caregiver should first encourage the woman to change positions (see Toolkit, Chapter 7, for positions for second stage), perhaps to a gravity-enhancing position. This often helps her to focus and push more effectively. Alternatively, the caregiver should instruct the woman to open her eyes and direct her gaze (and her bearing-down efforts) toward her vagina, and think about pressing the baby down and out. The woman may need frequent reminders to keep her eyes open. It may also help to remind her of her baby, that her baby is bringing her pain out of her body. We call this 'self-directed pushing', because the caregiver is helping the woman to direct her own bearing-down efforts.

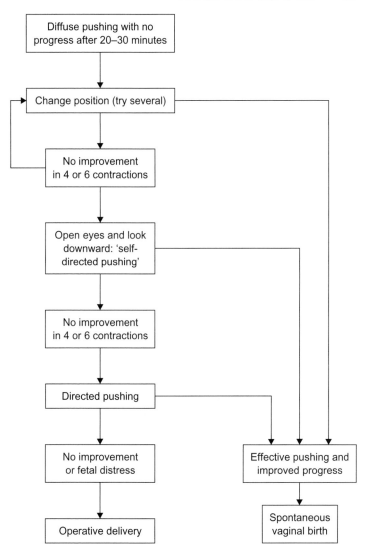

Chart 6.3 Diffuse pushing without progress.

These simple measures, opening her eyes and focusing on her baby moving down, usually result in progress without fetal distress or serious perineal damage. In those rare cases when these measures do not succeed, the caregiver may need to resort to encouraging her to do the prolonged breath-holding and maximal bearing down described earlier. If so, the caregiver should remember that the fetus usually tolerates the second stage better when the woman holds her breath and strains for less than seven seconds at a time[10,11,16,20]. If these measures do not succeed, consider emotional distress as a possible underlying cause. See pages 188–192 for measures to alleviate emotional dystocia.

If the woman has an epidural

Though epidural analgesia confers excellent pain relief most of the time, there are trade-offs involved which may increase both the length of the second stage and the need for instrumental delivery[21]. The search for the safest and most effective management of the second stage with an epidural is a subject of great interest for caregivers as well as for childbearing women, especially in areas where epidural use is extremely prevalent. Certainly, epidurals change the second stage for both the woman and her caregivers (Chart 6.4). Consider the following:

- Normally, the woman's pelvic floor provides a resilient platform on which the fetal head can rotate, and the muscles lining the pelvis also provide a resilient cushion that encourages rotation. Pressure on these muscles elicits a stretch response that plays an important role in the cardinal movements of descent (flexion, internal rotation, extension, and external rotation). With epidural analgesia, however, the pelvic floor muscles are anesthetized, resulting in a reduction of muscle tone, which may inhibit rotation of the fetal head[22]. This inhibition of the cardinal movements may help explain the increased need for instrumental deliveries with epidural analgesia[21]. When combined with maximal breath-holding and straining by the woman from the onset of the second stage, the likelihood of a difficult delivery due to a persistent malposition or a deep transverse arrest may be increased. Delaying pushing until the head is visible at the introitus or until the woman has an urge to push has been found to decrease the

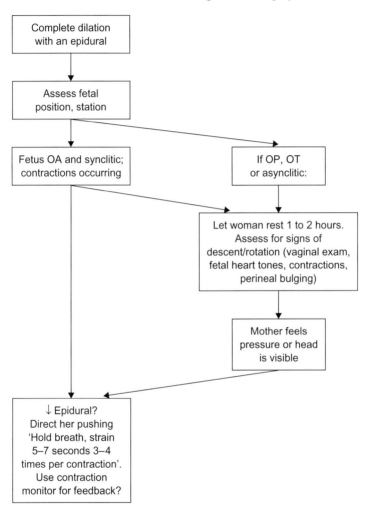

Chart 6.4 Delayed pushing with an epidural.

instrumental delivery rate[23], possibly by allowing more time for the fetus to gradually rotate and follow the path of least resistance down the birth canal. (Delayed pushing may provide little benefit if the fetus is already OA.) With anesthesia, the woman also lacks kinesthetic feedback to help her discover how to push effectively.

- An anesthetized woman is restricted to the few positions that she can assume without full sensation or use of her legs. These are usually limited to side-lying, supine, semi-sitting, sitting upright, or (in some cases with light anesthesia and good physical support) squatting, and hands and knees. Changing position usually requires assistance. Few studies of maternal positioning with an epidural exist, but it is an important area for investigation. One recent randomized controlled trial of women with epidurals in which passive descent (i.e. no pushing until the woman felt an urge to push or the fetal head was visible) was being used, compared outcomes with the lateral position versus supported sitting during the second stage[24]. The likelihood of instrumental delivery was more than twice as great in the women in the sitting position. This is the first trial to investigate position without prolonged bearing down efforts.

- Anesthesia may interfere with the usual spurt of endogenous oxytocin that is associated with pressure of the presenting part within the lower vagina[6–8]. Normally the pressure on the posterior vaginal wall or the pelvic floor signals the pituitary gland to release more oxytocin, resulting in stronger contractions, a greater urge to push, and more pressure on the pelvic floor. Anesthesia blocks this oxytocin-producing feedback loop, and progress is often impaired. Because of the reduced urge to push with an epidural, pushing requires a greater voluntary effort than pushing in response to an urge.

Some caregivers have tried to remedy the above problems by the following approaches to epidural management. The evidence for each is summarized:

- Using lower concentrations of the anesthetic when the epidural is first placed, possibly combining it with low dose narcotics, or using a combined spinal-epidural technique allow the woman more awareness and more motor control. Trials have found no difference in operative deliveries or need for oxytocin with these approaches, when compared to higher doses[25].

- Discontinuing or decreasing the dose of the epidural at the end of the first stage of labor is sometimes done, with the purpose of improving pelvic floor muscle tone, encouraging rotation, and reducing the need for instrumental delivery. A systematic review of trials of this technique found insufficient evidence of benefit, and inadequate pain relief. The numbers of women in the trials were quite small, and a large trial would provide stronger evidence on the real effect of discontinuing the epidural[26].

- As described above, delaying pushing for up to two hours, or until the fetal head is OA, or becomes visible at the vaginal outlet (when the labia are parted) may reduce the need for forceps rotation without risk to the newborn[23]. Evidence indicates that when pushing is delayed, thus avoiding forcing descent, the malpositioned fetus will often in time rotate and align well in the pelvis.

- Removing the time limit for second stage with an epidural improves the chances of a spontaneous delivery without risk to the neonate. The evidence supports this approach. Even if rotation and descent are slow, as long as fetus and woman are tolerating it well, many caregivers see no medical reason to intervene[11].

Pushing effectively with an epidural

Pushing with an epidural is often frustrating and ineffective, especially if the woman is unaware of an urge to push. The caregiver's urgent pleas for her to 'Push! Push!' along with a count to ten may make her feel that she cannot do it right. One way to help the woman push well and feel good about it is to use the electronic fetal monitor as a biofeedback device to encourage her efforts. By positioning him- or herself with both the monitor and the woman in view, the partner, doula, or nurse can watch the digital contraction indicator and instruct the woman when to begin bearing down (when the intensity rises about 30 mm Hg above baseline). He or she calls out the numbers as the contraction builds, then instructs her to bear down, and continues to call out the numbers, which will increase

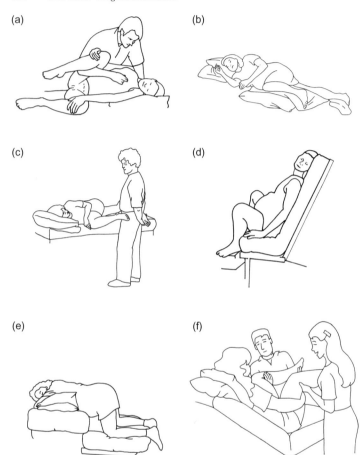

Fig. 6.2 a–h Pushing positions that may be used when women have epidurals. (a) Side-lying to push. (b) Semi-prone. (c) Side-lying lunge; (d) Semi-sitting. (e) Kneeling on foot of bed. (f) Semi-sitting, with people supporting the woman's legs. (g) Supine with leg supports. (h) Lap squatting.

(g)　　　　　　　　　　　　　　(h)

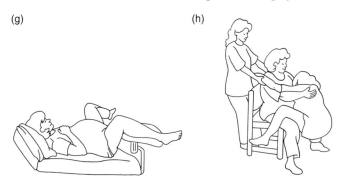

Fig. 6.2 (continued)

rapidly with her bearing-down effort, and which should last for five to seven seconds. Then the partner tells her to breathe 'for the baby' several times and to bear down again, repeating the numbers. ('Now bear down . . . That's it, 70, 73, 77, 84, 90! Go for 100! Great! You did it! Now breathe for the baby!')

This approach to bearing down emulates spontaneous bearing down, which results in better fetal oxygenation than prolonged and constant breath-holding and straining[11]. Chart 6.4 summarizes the instructions for delayed pushing with an epidural. If progress is slow, changing positions every 20 to 30 minutes often improves progress. Fig. 6.2a–h illustrates pushing positions that may be used when women have epidurals, depending on the density of the epidural block.

How long an active phase of second stage is too long?

Although some doctors and midwives limit the duration of second stage labor to two hours from complete dilation to birth, there is no scientific rationale for such an approach. The length of the second stage is not as important to a good outcome as the status of mother and baby during that time. Individualized care and careful assessment often allow more time for second stage with no compromise in the well-being of mother or baby[11]. An extensive review of the scientific literature on this issue concludes:

'There is no evidence to suggest that, when the second stage of labor is progressing and the condition of both woman and fetus is satisfactory, the imposition of any upper arbitrary limit on its duration is justified. Such limits should be discarded'[27].

A recent retrospective review of the effect of duration of second stage on fetal distress and maternal perinatal morbidity concluded that duration alone should not form the basis for decisions to intervene[28].

POSSIBLE ETIOLOGIES AND SOLUTIONS FOR SECOND-STAGE DYSTOCIA

The challenge for caregivers in a long second stage is to identify reasons for the slow progress and institute appropriate corrective measures. The choice of early interventions depends, to an extent, on the presumed etiology, although a trial and error approach is sometimes warranted.

Positions and other strategies for suspected occiput posterior (OP) or persistent occiput transverse (OT) fetuses

Fig. 6.3a–d illustrates abdominal and vaginal views of the OP and OT positions. As long as the woman is well supported and she has no musculoskeletal or medical problems, and her fetus is monitored, a wide variety of positions may be used to promote descent.

Why not the dorsal position?

Dorsal maternal positions tend to exacerbate fetal malpositions and deny the effects of gravity. See pages 119, 123, 184–186 and Chapter 7 for information on the disadvantages of supine positions. In some specific situations, however, the advantages of exaggerated lithotomy may outweigh the risks. (See Chapter 7, page 187.) For most women, the positions shown in Fig. 6.4a–f are more effective in promoting fetal rotation and descent, and may be more comfortable for the woman than the dorsal positions. Changing positions every 20 minutes (every five or six contractions) when progress is slow may help solve the problem. Even if the fetus cannot be rotated, these same measures may make a vaginal birth possible in a persistent OP or OT position.

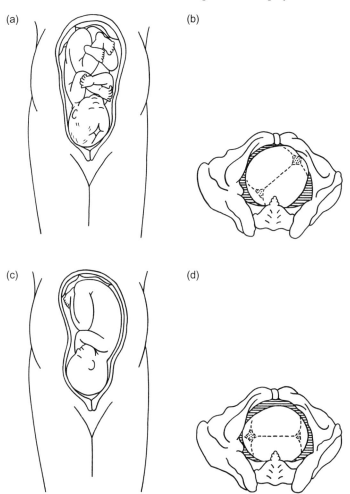

Fig. 6.3 (a) Right occiput posterior fetus, abdominal view. (b) Left occiput transverse fetus, abdominal view. (c) Right occiput posterior, fetus in synclitism, vaginal view. (d) Left occiput transverse fetus, vaginal view.

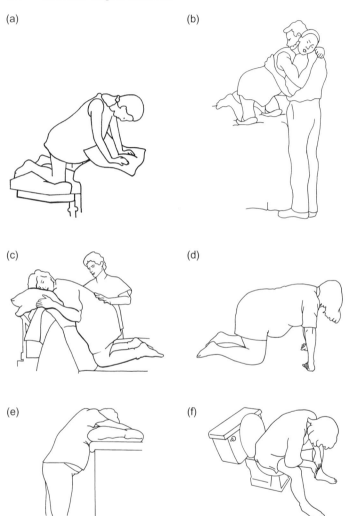

Fig. 6.4 a–f Pushing positions to promote rotation and descent
(a) Kneeling on foot of bed. (b) Kneeling, leaning on partner to push.
(c) Kneeling, leaning on the raised head of the bed. (d) Hands and knees.
(e) Standing, leaning on counter. (f) Sitting forward on toilet.

Differentiating between pushing positions and birth positions

Many maternal positions used to enhance progress would be awkward or uncomfortable for the caregiver during the actual birth. It may help to think of these as 'pushing positions', and to distinguish them from 'birth positions'. The woman may use a variety of pushing positions to bring the baby down, and then when the birth is imminent, assume a position that allows the attendant to see adequately, support the perineum, and 'catch' the baby without awkwardness or back strain.

Leaning forward while kneeling, standing, or sitting

These positions (Fig. 6.4a–f) take advantage of gravity to encourage rotation of the fetal trunk from posterior to anterior. Back pain, common with OP, is also relieved because the pressure of the fetal head on the sacrum is relieved. See the Toolkit, Chapter 7, for more information.

Squatting positions

Squatting positions utilize weight-bearing with hip abduction to widen the pelvic outlet, which may enlarge the space in the pelvic basin enough to promote rotation and descent. See Fig. 6.5a and b and Chapter 7, pages 218–225, for more information on squatting.

6

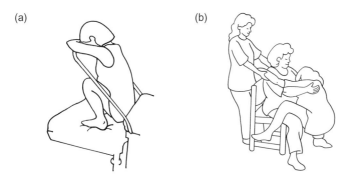

(a)   (b)

Fig. 6.5 (a) Squatting with bar. (b) Lap squatting.

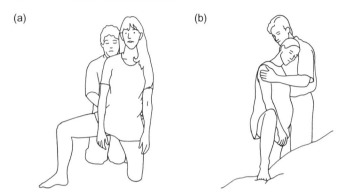

(a)   (b)

Fig. 6.6   (a) Asymmetrical kneeling. (b) Asymmetrical standing.

Asymmetrical positions

In asymmetrical positions the woman's legs are in different positions (for example, one knee up and one knee down). This changes the shape of the pelvis in ways that are different from 'symmetrical' positions such as squatting, and hands and knees. The pelvic joints on one side of the pelvis widen more than the joints on the other side. Sometimes the fetus is more likely to rotate with asymmetrical positions. See Fig. 6.6a and b, and pages 118 and 216–217 for more information on asymmetrical positions.

Lateral positions

For the woman who is exhausted or restricted to bed, side-lying (Fig. 6.7a) and the semi-prone (exaggerated Sims') positions are good alternatives to the dorsal or semi-sitting positions. If the fetus is thought to be OP, the woman should lie on:

- The same side as the posterior occiput if side-lying
- The side opposite the posterior or transverse occiput if in semi-prone (exaggerated Sims') (Fig. 6.7b)

See the explanation of the different effects of the side-lying and semi-prone positions in Chapter 5.

(a)

(b)

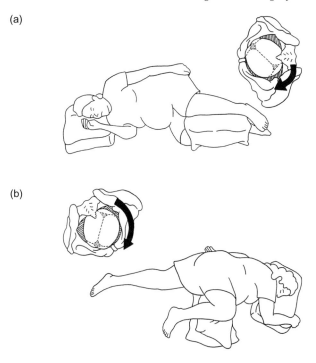

Fig. 6.7 (a) Woman with OP fetus in pure side-lying on the 'correct' side, with fetal back 'toward the bed'. If fetus is ROP, woman lies on her right side. Gravity pulls fetal occiput and trunk toward ROT. (b) Woman with OP fetus semi-prone on the 'correct' side, with fetal back 'toward the ceiling'. If fetus is ROP, the semi-prone woman lies on her left side. Gravity pulls fetal occiput and trunk toward ROT, then ROA.

Supported squat or 'dangle' positions

In these, the woman is supported under her arms, with minimal or no weight-bearing through her legs or feet (Fig. 6.8a–c). These are the only positions in which the woman is supported from her upper body. We propose the following mechanisms to explain how the dangle positions enhance the fetus's position.

The woman's own body weight lengthens her trunk by providing traction to her spinal column. This provides more vertical space for

(a)

(c)

(b)

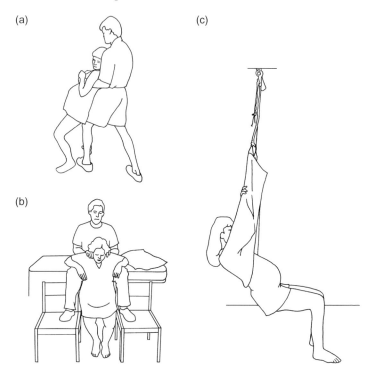

Fig. 6.8 Positions in which the woman is supported from her upper body. (a) Supported squat. (b) Dangle. (c) Dangle with birth sling.

6

the fetus to maneuver. Most second-stage positions require that the woman flex her trunk and neck, to add pressure to the fundus and promote descent of the fetus. However, this added pressure may not help if the head will not fit because it is asynclitic or deflexed. The dangle positions offer room for the head to reposition itself.

Furthermore, the dangle positions are free from external pressures on the pelvis, such as those that occur when the woman is sitting or lying down, or when her joints are stretched (e.g. when she squats or pulls her legs back). An absence of such external pressures, in cases where the fetal head appears to be 'stuck', may allow the pressure from the descending fetal head (and, presumably, fetal head movements) to change the shape of the pelvic basin as needed for the fetus to find the path of least resistance through the pelvis.

(a)

(b)

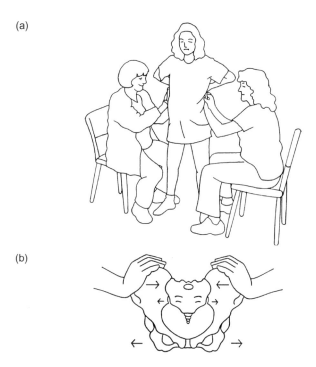

Fig. 6.9 (a) Positioning for pelvic press; (b) Detail of pelvic press.

Other strategies for malposition and back pain

The pelvic press may help in cases of deep transverse arrest, occiput posterior, or a 'tight fit' in the second stage, to increase midpelvic and outlet dimensions and aid fetal rotation and descent[29]. (See Fig. 6.9a and b and pages 241–242 for a description of the pelvic press.) This is not done with an epidural.

Please note that the pelvic press is not the same as the 'double hip squeeze'. The main difference between the two is the placement of the hands. In the pelvic press, the helper's hands are placed on the iliac crests; in the double hip squeeze, over the gluteal muscles on the buttocks. The pelvic press is used to enlarge the pelvic outlet in the second stage; the double hip squeeze is used to relieve back pain at any time in labor.

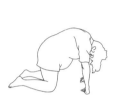

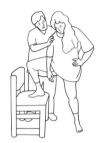

Fig. 6.10 Pelvic rocking, back rounded in flexion.

Fig. 6.11 Standing lunge.

A variety of movements may help rotate the fetus. See Chapter 7 for pelvic rocking (Fig. 6.10 and page 231), lunging (Fig. 6.11 and pages 216, 233–235), the kneeling lunge (Fig. 6.12), and slow dancing (Fig. 6.13 and page 236). Because extreme back pain often accompanies fetal malposition, measures to relieve this pain should be used as needed (Figs 6.14–6.20). If the back pain remains tolerable, the woman may have more patience to await fetal rotation and descent. See the Toolkit, Chapter 8, for instructions for these measures.

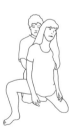

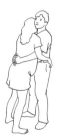

Fig. 6.12 Kneeling lunge.

Fig. 6.13 Slow dancing.

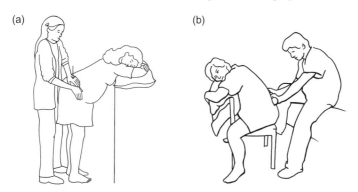

Fig. 6.14 (a) Counter-pressure. (b) Counter-pressure with tennis balls.

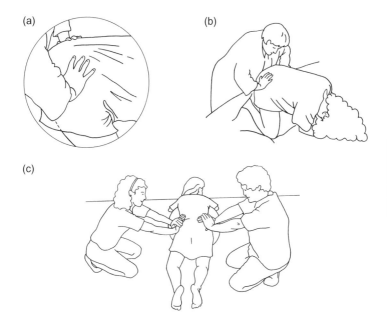

6

Fig. 6.15 More strategies for malposition and back pain. (a) Detail of double hip squeeze. (b) Double hip squeeze. (c) Double hip squeeze with two support people.

(a)

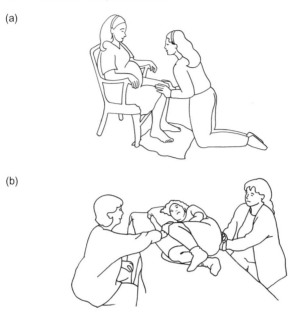

(b)

Fig. 6.16   (a) Knee press, woman seated. (b) Knee press, woman on her side.

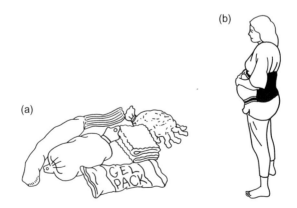

Fig. 6.17   (a) Heat and cold. (b) Strap-on cold pack.

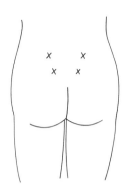

Fig. 6.18 Intradermal sterile water injection sites for back pain.

Fig. 6.19 TENS in use.

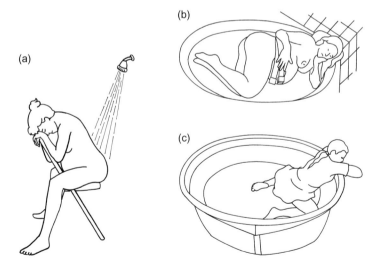

Fig. 6.20 Hydrotherapy for back pain: (a) Shower on woman's back to relieve back pain. (b) Side-lying in bath to relieve back pain. (c) Kneeling, leaning forward in birthing pool to relieve back pain.

Manual interventions to reposition the OP fetus

Manual rotation of a persistent occiput posterior is a technique described years ago by Hamlin[30], and in many subsequent obstetrics textbooks, including one recently by Davis[29]. Davis describes ways to disengage the fetal head slightly and rotate the head and trunk to anterior (or, if necessary, to direct OP) to facilitate descent (Chart 6.5).

Such techniques involve slightly dislodging the fetal head manually per vagina and rotating it to OA, or rotating the woman while holding the fetal head to keep it from rotating. Potential risks of such techniques include cord prolapse or compression, but the incidence of success and of risks has not been documented. It is beyond the scope of this book to describe such techniques as they are not used as 'early interventions'. The reader is referred to the references for further discussion.

Early interventions for suspected persistent asynclitism

Normally, at the onset of labor the fetal head is asynclitic (angled so that one parietal bone, located above the ear, is presenting), which facilitates entry of the head into the pelvic basin. This usually resolves spontaneously to synclitism as the fetus moves lower in the pelvis. (Fig. 6.21a–f show vaginal views of asynclitic and synclitic fetuses in OA, OP and OT.) However, persistent asynclitism in the second stage may interfere with flexion, rotation, molding and descent of the fetal head. A caput (swelling of soft tissue) often forms over one parietal bone.

Extra time and specific interventions encourage the fetus to shift into a more synclitic position. If the caregiver suspects persistent asynclitism, changing the woman's position may assist labor progress in three ways:

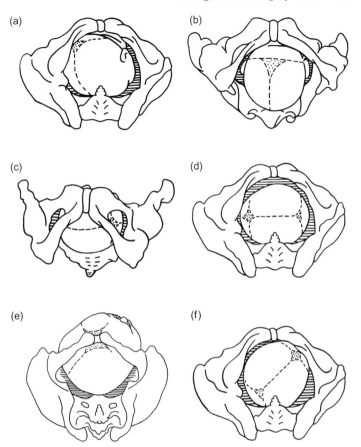

Fig. 6.21 (a) Asynclitic fetus in occiput anterior. (b) Occiput anterior in synclitism. (c) Asynclitic fetus in occiput transverse. (d) Occiput transverse in synclitism. (e) Asynclitic fetus in right occiput posterior. (f) Right occiput posterior in synclitism.

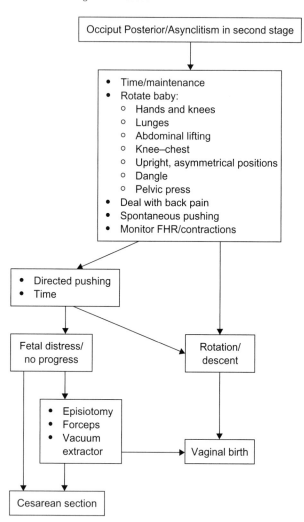

Chart 6.5   Occiput posterior/asynclitism in second stage.

(1) Shifting the woman may shift the fetus' weight so its position resolves.

(2) Changing the woman's position may alter the shape of her pelvis slightly, allowing more room for the angle of the fetal head to shift.

(3) Having the woman take a position that elongates her torso (i.e. the dangle and supported squat) may give the fetus room enough to 'wiggle' out of asynclitism. See pages 168–169 for a complete explanation.

Positions and movements for persistent asynclitism in second stage

In general, the same positions and movements, and back pain relief techniques, pages 162–174, for persistent OP/OT are useful when the fetus seems to be in a persistent asynclitic position. (See the Toolkit, Chapter 7, for information on specifics.) Specifically, pelvic press, and the dangle and supported squat positions may be especially helpful when the fetus is thought to be asynclitic during the second stage. Success with these positions will be influenced by the degree of engagement of the fetal head and the fit between fetal head and woman's pelvis. These techniques merit further study, since the advantages ascribed to them are theoretical and observational[31].

Manual repositioning of the asynclitic fetal head

Doctors and midwives (not maternity nurses or doulas) sometimes try to correct asynclitism manually by dislodging the fetal head and repositioning it so that the sagittal suture line is centered[30]. The technique requires further study of effectiveness and safety.

6

If cephalo-pelvic disproportion (CPD) or macrosomia is suspected

A variety of factors may contribute to a slow second stage and create doubt whether the baby will fit through the woman's pelvis. These include the size and shape of the fetal head, the size and shape of the woman's pelvis, the position of the fetus, and the woman's ability to move around during labor.

The influence of time on CPD

Many suspected cases of CPD actually involve fetuses who are subtly malpositioned (asynclitic, deflexed, occiput transverse or posterior), who will fit well through the pelvis once the malposition has been resolved. The shape of the woman's pelvis is also a consideration. The woman may need to try pushing in a variety of positions to find the ones that optimize descent. Resolving problems of position or fit often requires extra time.

Many large fetal heads will mold and fit safely through the pelvis, but molding takes time. In the absence of fetal or maternal distress, time can be an ally, not an enemy, in allowing labor progress to take place.

Some midwives and doctors have strict expectations for an acceptable rate of progress in descent. If progress falls behind the expected rate, they initiate interventions such as oxytocin, fundal pressure, episiotomy, forceps, vacuum extraction, or cesarean delivery. Others, however, prefer to exercise patience and less aggressive interventions as long as the fetus appears to be doing well and the woman is willing and able to continue.

Note: Ultrasound predictions of fetal size

Ultrasound measurements of fetal weight and head size are not always reliable. For babies weighing over 4000 g (8 lb 13 oz), they can err by 10% (almost a pound) in either direction[32]. Furthermore, even accurate estimates of fetal head size and weight do not predict the capacity of the fetal head or the pelvis to mold to accommodate safe passage of the fetus.

Positions for 'possible CPD' second stage

Because 'suspected CPD' often results from fetal malpositions, rather than from a true excess of the diameters of the fetal head over the diameters of the pelvic basin, it makes sense to encourage the woman to try positions and movements that might resolve an OP, OT, or asynclitic position (Figs 6.22–6.30). See also Chapter 7 for a discussion of these positions and movements.

Positions for 'possible CPD' second stage, cont'd

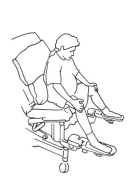

Fig. 6.22 Sitting upright to push.

Fig. 6.23 Pushing on a birthing stool (adapted from a photo of the DeBY Birth Support).

(a)

(b)

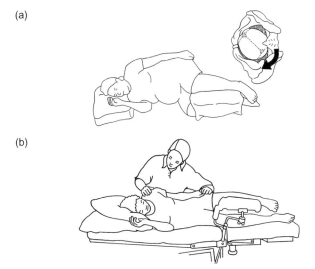

Fig. 6.24 (a) and (b) Woman with an OP fetus in pure side-lying on the 'correct' side, with fetal back 'toward the bed'. If fetus is ROP, woman lies on her right side. Gravity pulls fetal head and trunk toward OT.

Positions for 'possible CPD' second stage, cont'd

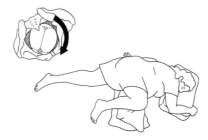

Fig. 6.25 Woman semi-prone on the 'correct' side, with fetal back 'toward the ceiling'. If fetus is ROP, the semi-prone woman lies on her left side. Gravity pulls fetal head and trunk toward ROT, then ROA.

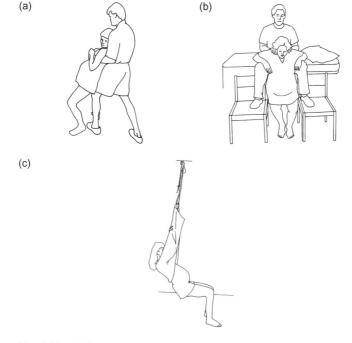

Fig. 6.26   (a) Supported squat. (b) Dangle. (c) Dangle with a birth sling.

Positions for 'possible CPD' second stage, cont'd

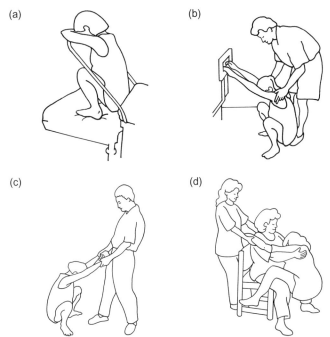

Fig. 6.27 (a) Squatting with a bar. (b) Squatting with bed rail. (c) Partner squat. (d) Lap squat, three person.

Toilet-sitting and hydrotherapy may also enhance progress (Figs 6.28 and 6.29).

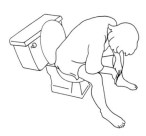

Fig. 6.28 Sitting forward on toilet.

Positions for 'possible CPD' second stage, cont'd

(a)

(b)

(c)

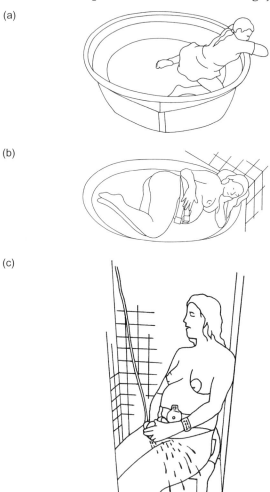

Fig. 6.29   (a) Woman in a birth pool. (b) Woman in bath, with telemetry monitors. (c) Woman in shower, with telemetry monitors.

Encourage movements that adapt pelvic size and shape and encourage fetal descent (Figs 6.30 and 6.31). See page 22 for notes on movement and why it helps.

Note: To master the technique of the lunge, see the instructions on pages 222–224, and 233–235 before teaching it to the woman in labor.

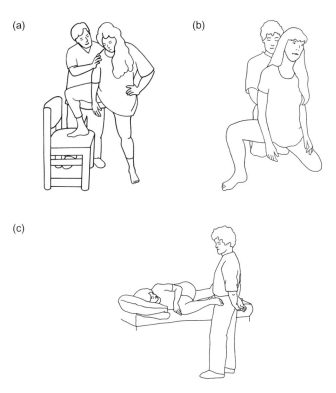

(a)

(b)

(c)

Fig. 6.30   (a) Standing lunge. (b) Kneeling lunge. (c) Side-lying lunge.

Positions for 'possible CPD' second stage, cont'd

(a)   (b)

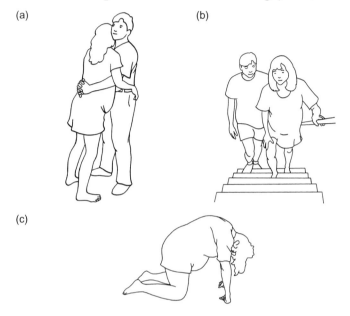

(c)

Fig. 6.31 (a) Slow dancing. (b) Stair climbing. (c) Pelvic rocking, back rounded in flexion.

The use of dorsal positions

Dorsal positions are the most commonly suggested positions for the second stage today. In fact, many women spend the entire second stage in a dorsal or semi-sitting position (Fig. 6.32a–d), even though they would probably use a variety of positions, including upright ones, if given a choice[18]. Though dorsal positions are convenient for caregivers to view the perineum easily, and to perform vaginal exams, episiotomy, vacuum extraction, and forceps, there are some problems associated with these positions. The woman's body weight on the bed creates pressure on her sacrum and coccyx, which reduces the antero-posterior diameter of the pelvic outlet[33–34]. Compare parts (a) and (b) of Fig. 6.33. The effects of gravity in promoting descent are lost with supine or any recumbent positions[33–34].

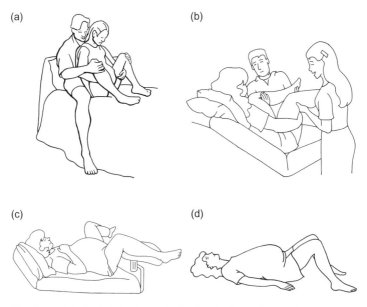

Fig. 6.32 (a) Semi-sitting to push. (b) Semi-sitting with people supporting the woman's legs. (c) Supine with leg supports. (d) Supine, hips and knees flexed.

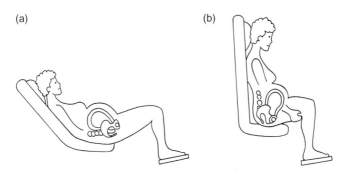

Fig. 6.33 (a) Woman reclining. Adapted from reference 33. (b) Woman upright. Adapted from reference 33.

Maternal supine hypotension is caused by the weight of the uterus on the inferior vena cava and aorta, which leads to a reduction in venous return and cardiac output. The fetus may then experience hypoxia due to the concomitant decrease in blood flow to the placenta and resulting reduction in oxygen supply to the fetus, especially if combined with prolonged breath-holding and maximal straining[11]. Besides supine hypotension, the weight of the uterus along the spinal column reduces the angle of the uterus with the spine, resulting in poor alignment of the fetus with the pelvis[33] (Fig. 2.2, page 23).

With persistent OP, persistent asynclitism, or other malpositions, the woman should be encouraged to do most of her pushing in positions other than supine or semi-sitting. It is ironic that two widely prescribed practices for second stage, prolonged breath-holding and straining, and the supine position, are at least partly responsible for the frequently observed fetal bradycardias and prolonged second stage that have led caregivers to believe that the duration of the second stage must be curtailed. The further irony is that if laboring women were encouraged to behave instinctually, they would not lie on their backs, nor would they use prolonged breath-holding and straining; thus, much of the worrisome 'fetal distress' in the second stage would not occur.

Use of the exaggerated lithotomy position

Notwithstanding what was stated above, there are occasions when one particular dorsal position, the exaggerated lithotomy (McRoberts') position, may succeed in promoting descent when other positions do not. When the woman has been unable to bring her baby beneath the pubic symphysis in any other position, this problem may in some cases be resolved by having the woman lie flat on her back with her knees drawn back (by herself or others) so that her buttocks are lifted slightly off the bed, and her hips are in a very flexed, abducted position (Figs 6.34a and b). This position passively rotates the pubic arch upward toward the mother's head and brings the pelvic inlet perpendicular to the maximum expulsive force[33,35,36].

(a) (b)

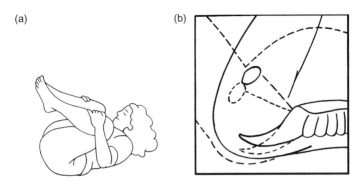

Fig. 6.34 (a) Exaggerated lithotomy position. (b) Exaggerated lithotomy (detail).

Such a position may facilitate the passage of the fetal head beneath the pubic arch. In persistent delays in descent this benefit may outweigh the disadvantages of supine hypotension and loss of any gravity advantage. Such a position is combined with maximal breath-holding and straining. It is worth trying when operative delivery is anticipated.

A note of caution: Those who are supporting the woman's legs in the exaggerated lithotomy position must exercise particular caution not to pull her legs too far out to the sides or too far up to her shoulders. This can cause damage to her pubic symphysis, sacroiliac joints, or hip joints or it may cause nerve damage[37]. This is especially true if the mother cannot feel these joints, as with an epidural.

6

Shoulder dystocia

Shoulder dystocia is defined as a birth requiring extra maneuvers to deliver the fetus after the head is born[38]. One shoulder is caught on the mother's pubic symphysis, and internal rotation and descent are delayed. Shoulder dystocia requires quick thinking and calm, effective management, at a time when the caregiver may be frightened or anxious. Specific maneuvers, such as McRoberts' position, pressure just above the woman's pubic symphysis, rolling the woman onto hands and knees (Gaskin maneuver), placing a hand in the vagina to rotate the baby's shoulder, and others, require knowledge and skill. Most resolve quickly with such actions. Because treatment of shoulder dystocia is beyond the scope of this book, we refer the reader to authoritative textbooks and articles for more explanation of techniques for correcting a shoulder dystocia[38].

If contractions are inadequate

If contraction intensity and frequency decrease during the second stage, the possible causes should be considered. They are likely to be the same as those discussed in Chapter 5. Immobility, medications, dehydration, and maternal exhaustion are all possible causes. Contractions might be improved by such measures as changing positions; allowing the medications or epidural to wear off (if the woman can tolerate it); breast stimulation; hydration; allowing the woman to avoid voluntary or forceful pushing for a number of contractions; or immersion in water. These are almost the same measures as those suggested for inadequate contractions during the active phase of first stage. Please read pages 123–131 for detailed explanations of these possible causes and solutions for inadequate contractions.

If emotional dystocia is suspected

Emotional distress sometimes underlies a lack of progress in the second stage. Much of the information in Chapters 2 and 5, on the physiology of emotional dystocia and on measures to alleviate it during the first stage of labor, also applies to the second stage.

The essence of coping during the second stage of labor

Before discussing other factors that may trigger emotional distress, let us review what 'coping well' during the second stage means.

When the second stage begins, the woman, if undisturbed and unrestricted, becomes more aware of her surroundings, alert, and energetic. As her reflexive urge to push intensifies, it guides her to bear down and find a position that feels right. As the baby moves down the vaginal canal, she may temporarily 'hold back' (tense her perineum, fearing the stretching feeling). As her body's strong urges take over she lets go, releasing her pelvic floor and her attempts to control the process. She may grunt, moan, or even bellow with her contractions as she instinctively moves into different positions. The 3Rs (pages 135–136) no longer apply.

The caregiver's role when a woman is coping in this way is to monitor the fetus' and mother's well-being as unobtrusively as possible, provide encouragement and reassurance as needed, and accommodate and support her instinctive behaviors as much as possible. There are many safe and effective positions and ways of bearing down. As long as mother and baby are tolerating the second stage and some progress is being made, there is no reason to intervene. (When it is clear that the baby will be born soon, it may be necessary to ask the mother to adopt a position in which the clinical caregiver has adequate access.)

In summary, 'coping well' during the second stage includes grunting and bearing down reflexively with the urge to push (even bellowing at times), breathing as desired between bearing down efforts, and moving into positions that feel right. These behaviors are signs of normal coping, not signs of distress.

Signs of emotional distress in second stage

- Verbal or facial expressions of fear
- Crying or panic
- Inability to get beyond holding back to releasing the pelvic floor – previous trauma, holding her legs together, or diffuse pushing (pages 153–156)
- Begging the caregiver to take the baby out or to 'knock' her out with drugs
- Desperation, inability to follow caregiver's suggestions

Triggers of emotional distress unique to the second stage

These factors might trigger emotional distress and interfere with the woman's ability to cope during the second stage:

- Fatigue or exhaustion, which can lead to hopelessness or anxiety.
- The intense sensations of second stage or of manual stretching of the vagina. These sensations may be especially frightening if the woman has been sexually abused in the past, as they may trigger flashbacks to the abuse.
- Fear of behaving inappropriately or offensively (making noise, passing stool while pushing).
- The immediacy of the birth and the responsibility of parenting the child, especially if her own parents were dysfunctional, or she has relinquished a child for adoption, or had a child removed from her care.
- Fear for the baby's well-being, especially if a sibling or a previous child died around birth or had another adverse outcome.
- The loss of privacy, sense of modesty when surrounded by strangers watching her perineum.
- Previous cesarean during second stage.
- Thoughtless or unkind treatment by loved ones or caregiver during labor.

One common response to such fears in the second stage is extreme tension in the pelvic floor as if to deter the fetus's descent, while pushing. The woman may be pushing hard, but not effectively. Sometimes she actually contracts her pelvic floor muscles and buttocks as she pushes with her diaphragm and abdominal muscles. Tension in the perineum and constriction of the anus while pushing indicate that the woman is holding back. (It is important not to confuse this excessive and prolonged pelvic tension with the normal confusion many women have when they first begin to push. It is normal for women to experiment a bit in order to discover how to push effectively. This is particularly true for women who do not initially have a strong urge to push. In such cases, it may be best for them to rest and await a stronger urge to push.)

If a woman exhibits 'diffuse pushing' (see pages 153–156) and does not benefit from the measures to improve her bearing-down efforts, consider the possibility of emotional dystocia.

Whatever fears or anxieties cause the woman to hold back, she probably cannot simply 'snap out of it'. However, those around her may be able to address and alleviate her fears. The measures described in Chapter 4 may help, along with the following:

- Encourage the woman to express her feelings. Ask her, 'What was going through your mind during that last contraction?' Listen to her, acknowledge and validate her concerns, and try to give appropriate reassurance, encouragement, or information and suggestions. Often, all the woman needs is a chance to express her concerns. She needs to know that she is being heard, that her fears are normal, and that she will get through this event. Even normal events can be very troublesome to an anxious woman.

- Sometimes, when it is clear to everyone including the woman, that there is a delay, asking her why she thinks labor has slowed down, reveals useful information. Answers such as, 'I can't push right', or, 'The baby doesn't want to come out', might indicate emotional dystocia.

- Provide appropriate information. For example, if the woman is afraid of having a bowel movement as she pushes (and it is too late for her to go to the bathroom), she can be reassured that passing stool indicates that she is pushing effectively, that this is a common event, that any fecal material will be quickly wiped away and disposed of. In fact, this is one of many good reasons to apply warm compresses to the perineum at this time – to be able to unobtrusively remove stool.

- If she is afraid she will 'rip' or split apart while pushing, reassure her that, by relaxing her perineum or letting the baby come, it actually stretches better and a tear is less likely. Also, unless there is a good reason not to do so, let her try a few contractions without pushing. 'Let's try breathing through this next one', so that she feels she has some options during this frightening time.

6

- Give the woman time to adjust to the intense sensations and emotions of second stage. Avoid creating a sense of rushing. There is usually no need for the caregiver to raise his or her voice.

- Encourage the woman to relax her perineum between contractions and let it bulge during contractions. The application of hot compresses (washcloths soaked in hot water, wrung out) to the perineum often feels good and promotes relaxation. The compresses should not be too hot for the person applying them to hold comfortably in his or her hand. Encourage the woman to push as if she is blowing up an imaginary balloon, or as if she were trying to urinate rapidly. Pushing in this manner sometimes causes the pelvic floor to bulge, which the caregiver can see. If she seems reluctant to sustain a bearing-down effort and she is not making progress, advise her to 'Push to the pain, and right through it. It will feel better when you push through it.'

- Have the woman try pushing while sitting on the toilet. If she is worried about passing stool, the toilet is a reassuring place to be. Toilet-sitting also elicits the conditioned response of releasing the pelvic floor. Whoever is responsible for the woman's care can monitor what the woman is feeling. If the woman feels that the baby is coming, she will need to move to a more appropriate delivery site.

If the woman is pushing in a 'diffuse' manner, see pages 153–156.

CONCLUSION

The conduct of second stage of labor has long been guided by principles of speed and convenience for the care provider. Many practices, such as early maximal bearing down, immobility, the dorsal or another horizontal position, and a time limit actually interfere with progress, and frequently necessitate such interventions as IV oxytocin, forceps, vacuum extractor, episiotomy, or cesarean delivery. In this chapter, we present an approach designed to foster optimal progress, and implement simple interventions in order to prevent serious cases of failed progress.

REFERENCES

1. Simkin, P. (1984) Active and physiologic management of second stage: a review and hypothesis. In: *Episiotomy and the Second Stage of Labor* (eds S. Kitzinger & P. Simkin). ICEA, Minneapolis.

2. Simkin, P. (2001) *The Birth Partner*, 2nd edn. Harvard Common Press, Boston.

3. Kitzinger, S. (2003) *The Complete Book of Pregnancy and Childbirth*. Alfred A. Knopf, New York.

4. Friedman, E.A. (1978) Normal labor. In: *Labor: Clinical Evaluation and Management*, 2nd edn. Appleton Century Crofts, New York.

5. Cohen, W.R. & Friedman, E.A. (1983) Dysfunctional labor. In: *Management of Labor*. University Park Press, Baltimore.

6. Vasicka, A., Kumaresan, P., Han, G.S. & Kumaresan, M. (1978) Plasma oxytocin in initiation of labor. *American Journal of Obstetrics and Gynecology*, **130** (3), 263–73.

7. Fuchs, A.R., Romero, R., Keefe, D., Parra, M., Oyarzun, E. & Behnke, E. (1991) Oxytocin secretion and human parturition: pulse frequency and duration increase during spontaneous labor in women. *American Journal of Obstetrics and Gynecology*, **165** (5, Part 1), 1515–23.

8. Rahm, V., Hallgren, A., Hogberg, H., Hurtig, I. & Odlind, V. (2002) Plasma oxytocin levels in women during labor with or without epidural analgesia: a prospective study. *Acta Obstetrica Gynecologica Scandinavica*, **81**, 1033–9.

9. Beynon, C.L. (1957) The normal second stage of labour: a plea for reform in its conduct. *Journal of Obstetrics and Gynaecology British Commonwealth*, **64** (6), 815–20.

10. Enkin, M., Keirse, M., Neilsen, J., *et al.* (2000) Monitoring the progress of labour, Chapter 31. In: *A Guide to Effective Care in Pregnancy and Childbirth*, 3rd edn. Oxford University Press, Oxford.

11. Roberts, J. (2002) The 'push' for evidence: management of the second stage. *Journal of Midwifery and Womens' Health*, **47**, 2–15.10.

12. BMA/RPSGB (1997) *British National Formulary*. British Medical Association and The Royal Pharmaceutical Society of Great Britain, Number 33, Pharmaceutical Press, London.

13. Rosevear, S. & Stirrat, G. (1996) *The Handbook of Obstetric Management*. Blackwell Scientific, Oxford.

14. Sinclair, C. (2004) *A Midwife's Handbook*. Saunders, St Louis.

15. Bing, E. (1994) Personal communication.

16. Aldrich, C.J., D'Antona, D., Spencer, J.A.D., *et al.* (1995) The effect of maternal pushing on fetal cerebral oxygenation and blood volume during the second stage of labour. *British Journal of Obstetrics and Gynaecology*, **102**, 448–53.

6

17. Schaffer, J., Bloom, B., Casey, D., McIntire, M., Nihira, K. & Leveno, K. (2005) A randomized trial of the effects of coached vs. uncoached maternal pushing during the second stage of labor on postpartum pelvic floor structure and function. *American Journal of Obstetrics and Gynecology*, **192**, 1692–6.

18. Carlson, J.M., Diehl, J.A., Sachtleben-Murray, M., McRae, M., Fenwick, L. & Friedman, E.A. (1986) Maternal position during parturition in normal labor. *Obstetrics and Gynecology*, **68** (4), 443–7.

19. Fuller, B.F., Roberts, J.E. & McKay, S. (1993) Acoustical analysis of maternal sounds during the second stage of labor. *Applied Nursing Research*, **6**, 7–13.

20. Caldeyro-Barcia, R. (1986) Influence of maternal bearing-down efforts during second stage on fetal well-being. In: *Episiotomy and the Second Stage of Labor* (eds S. Kitzinger & P. Simkin). ICEA, Minneapolis.

21. Howell, C. (1999) Epidural versus non-epidural analgesia for pain relief in labour. *The Cochrane Database of Systematic Reviews*, Issue 3. Art. No.: CD000331. DOI: 10.10022/14651858.CD000331.

22. Bonica, J.J., Miller, F.C. & Parmley, T.H. (1995) Anatomy and physiology of the forces of parturition. In: *Principles and Practice of Obstetric Analgesia and Anesthesia*, 2nd edn (eds J.J. Bonica & J.S. McDonald). Williams & Wilkins, Philadelphia.

23. Fraser, W., Marcoux, S., Krauss, I., Douglas, J., Goulet, C. & Boulvain, M. (2002) Multicenter, randomized, controlled trial of delayed pushing for nulliparous women in the second stage of labor with continuous epidural analgesia. The PEOPLE (Pushing Early or Pushing Late with Epidural) Study. *Obstetrics and Gynecology*, **99**, 409–18.

24. Downe, S., Gerrett, D. & Renfrew, M. (2004) A prospective randomized trial on the effect of position in the passive second stage of labour on birth outcome in nulliparous women using epidural analgesia. *Midwifery*, **20**, 157–68.

25. Hughes, D., Simmons, S., Brown, J. & Cyna, A. (2003) Combined spinal-epidural versus epidural analgesia in labour. *The Cochrane Database of Systematic Reviews*, Issue 4. Atr. No.: CD003401.nDOI: 10.1002/14651858.CD003401.

26. Torvaldsen, S., Roberts, C., Bell, J. & Raynes-Greenow, C. (2004) Discontinuation of epidural analgesia late in labour for reducing the adverse delivery outcomes associated with epidural analgesia. *The Cochrane Database of Systematic Reviews*, Issue 4. Art. No.: CD00457.pub2. DOI: 10.1002/14651858.CD004457.pub2.

27. Enkin, M., Keirse, M., Neilsen, J., *et al.* (2000) The second stage of labour, Chapter 32, page 298. In: *A Guide to Effective Care in Pregnancy and Childbirth*, 3rd edn. Oxford University Press, Oxford.

6

28. Janni, W., Schiessl, B., Peschers, U., *et al.* (2002) The prognostic impact of a prolonged second stage of labor on maternal and fetal outcome. *Acta Obstetrica Gynecologica Scandinavica*, **81**, 214–21.

29. Davis, E. (1997) *Heart and Hands: A Caregiver's Guide to Pregnancy and Birth*, 3rd edn. Celestial Arts, Berkeley.

30. Hamlin, R.H.J. (1959) *Stepping Stones to Labour Ward Diagnosis*. Rigby Ltd, Adelaide.

31. Simkin, P. (2003) Maternal positions and pelves revisited. *Birth*, **30**, 130–32.

32. Dudley, N. (2005) A systematic review of the ultrasound estimation of fetal weight. *Ultrasound in Obstetrics and Gynecology*, 25, 80–9.

33. Fenwick, L. & Simkin, P. (1987) Maternal position to prevent or alleviate dystocia in labor. *Clinical Obstetrics and Gynecology*, **30**, 83–9.

34. Michel, S., Rake, A., Treiber, K., *et al.* (2002) MR pelvimetry: effect of birthing position on pelvic bony dimensions. *American Journal of Roentgenology*, **179**, 1063–7.

35. Gherman, R., Tramont, J., Muffley, P. & Goodwin, T. (2000) Analysis of McRoberts' maneuver by X-ray pelvimetry. *Obstetrics and Gynecology*, **95**, 43–7.

36. Sweet, B.R. & Tiran, D. (eds) (1997) *Mayes' Midwifery*. Baillière Tindall, London.

37. Health, T. & Gherman, R. (1999) Symphyseal separation, sacroiliac joint dislocation, transient lateral femoral cutaneous neuropathy associated with McRoberts' maneuver. A case report. *Journal of Reproductive Medicine*, **44** (10), 902–4.

38. Baxley, E. & Gobbo, R. (2004) Shoulder dystocia. *American Family Physician*, **69**, 1707–1714.

6

Chapter 7

The Labor Progress Toolkit: Part 1. Maternal Positions and Movements

Maternal positions, 197
Side-lying positions, 198
The 'side-lying lunge', 202
Semi-sitting, 203
Sitting upright, 205
Sitting leaning forward with support, 207
Standing, leaning forward, 208
Kneeling, leaning forward with support, 210
Hands and knees, 212
Open knee–chest position, 213
Closed knee–chest position, 215
Asymmetrical upright (standing, kneeling, sitting) positions, 216
Squatting, 218
Supported squatting positions, 220
Half squatting, lunging and swaying, 222
Lap squatting, 224
Exaggerated lithotomy (McRoberts' position), 226
Supine, 228
Rope pull, 229
Maternal movements, 231
Pelvic rocking (also called pelvic tilt) and other movements of the pelvis, 231
The lunge, 233
Walking or stair climbing, 235
Slow dancing, 236
Abdominal stroking, 238
Abdominal lifting, 239
The pelvic press, 241
Other rhythmic movements, 243
References, 244

This Toolkit, which consists of Chapters 7 (Maternal Positions and Movements) and 8 (Comfort Measures), contains descriptions of numerous techniques for enhancing labor progress and maintaining comfort in both the first and second stages.

Many of these techniques are designed to improve the biomechanical forces of labor: the powers, passage, and passenger. They include such techniques as the woman's use of her own body; the use of props to support the woman in particular positions or movements; and the use of pressure or physical support by another person.

Many techniques are designed to reduce pain and enhance relaxation without using pain medications. When pain is reduced, the woman's tolerance of a prolonged labor is improved, which allows more time for the use of primary interventions. Without drugs, there are fewer, if any, side effects that might interfere with labor progress or adversely affect woman or baby.

Other techniques that reduce anxiety, fear, and distress may improve labor progress by decreasing maternal catecholamine production. Increased catecholamine production sometimes results in slowing of uterine contractions as well as fetal stress. Women who experience less anxiety and fear have lower catecholamine levels.

MATERNAL POSITIONS

This section contains descriptions of positions and specific features of each. We have arranged the positions in categories. The positions in each category cause similar physical changes. For example:

- Semi-sitting and side-lying positions are restful and gravity neutral. They may help an exhausted woman save her energy, especially if she has been up and walking for a long period. Also, if progress is rapid, neutralizing gravity may slow the labor to a more manageable pace.

- Upright positions take advantage of gravity to apply the presenting part to the cervix, improve the quality of the contractions, and enhance the descent of the fetus[1-2].

- Positions in which the woman leans forward tend to enhance fetal rotation and reduce back pain[3-6].

7

- Asymmetrical positions, in which the woman elevates one leg, change the shape of the pelvis, enhance rotation, and reduce back pain.

- The exaggerated lithotomy position, used for several contractions in the second stage, may facilitate the passage of a 'stuck baby' beneath the pubic symphysis.

- Dorsal positions tend to cause supine hypotension and increase back pain. Contractions are more frequent and painful, yet less likely to improve labor progress[1].

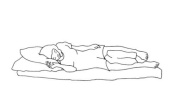

Fig. 7.1   Side-lying.   **Fig. 7.2**   Side-lying with leg in leg rest.

Side-lying positions

When

During first and second stages.

How

For pure side-lying: Woman lies on side with both hips and knees flexed and a pillow between her legs, or with her upper leg raised and supported (Figs 7.1–7.3).

For semi-prone or exaggerated Sims': Woman lies on side with lower arm behind (or in front of) her trunk, her lower leg extended, and her upper leg flexed more than 90° and supported by one or two pillows. She rolls partly toward her front (Figs 7.4–7.5). See below for information on which side the woman should lie on.

What these positions do

- Allow tired women to rest.

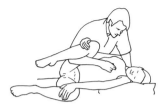

Fig. 7.3   Side-lying to push.

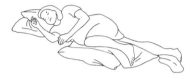

Fig. 7.4   Semi-prone, lower arm forward.

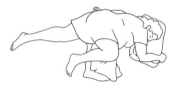

Fig. 7.5   Semi-prone, lower arm behind.

- Are safe if pain medications have been used.
- Are gravity neutral (can be used with a very rapid first or second stage).
- May relieve hemorrhoids.
- May resolve fetal heart rate problems, if due to cord compression or supine hypotension.
- Help lower high blood pressure (especially the left lateral positions).
- May promote progress when alternated with walking.
- Avoid pressure on sacrum (unlike sitting and supine positions).
- In second stage, because there is no pressure on the sacrum (as there is with sitting) these positions allow posterior movement of the sacrum as the fetus descends.
- May enhance rotation of an occiput posterior (OP) baby.

7

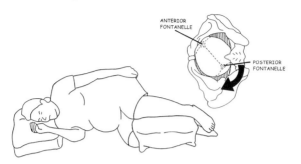

Fig. 7.6   Woman in pure side-lying on the 'correct' side, with fetal back 'toward the bed'. If fetus is ROP, woman lies on her right side. Gravity pulls fetal occiput and trunk toward ROT.

Note: Gravity effects are different when a woman is in pure side-lying or semi-prone.

If side-lying, the woman with an OP fetus should lie on the same side as the fetal occiput and back ('baby's back toward bed', Fig. 7.6). This helps shift the fetus from OP to OT. Ask the woman with an OP fetus to lie on the same side as the occiput for 15–30 minutes, to encourage rotation from OP to OT; then ask her to change to kneeling and leaning forward for 15–30 minutes (to encourage rotation from OT to occiput anterior). As can be seen in Fig. 7.7, lying on the side opposite the fetal occiput actually utilizes gravity to take the fetus into direct OP.

If the woman is semi-prone ('exaggerated Sims''), she should lie on the side opposite the fetal occiput ('baby's back toward ceiling', Fig. 7.8) for at least 15–30 minutes. In this position, her pelvis is rotated so that the pubis is pointing more toward the bed than with straight side-lying. This alters the effects of gravity so that the fetal trunk is encouraged to rotate to transverse and then to anterior.

When to use side-lying positions

- As long as labor continues to progress well and the woman wants it.
- When supine hypotension occurs.

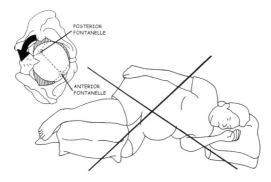

Fig. 7.7 Woman in pure side-lying on the 'wrong' (left) side for an ROP fetus. Fetal back is toward the ceiling. Gravity pulls fetal occiput and trunk toward OP.

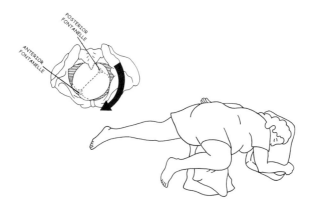

Fig. 7.8 Woman with OP fetus in semi-prone on the 'correct' side, with fetal back 'toward the ceiling'. If fetus is ROP, the semi-prone woman lies on left side. Gravity pulls the fetal occiput and trunk toward ROT, then ROA.

7

- When the woman has been given narcotics or an epidural.
- When the woman has pregnancy-induced hypertension.
- When the woman finds it comfortable in first or second stage.
- When the woman is tired.
- In second stage, if hemorrhoids are painful in dorsal positions.
- In a rapid second stage, to neutralize gravity effect.

When not to use side-lying positions

- When the woman refuses, due to increased pain or preference for another position. However, if it is explained that this position may improve labor progress, the woman may be willing to try it.
- When a gravity advantage is needed to aid descent, especially if second stage progress has slowed.
- When she has been in side-lying for more than an hour without progress.

The 'side-lying lunge'

When

During first and second stages.

How

With the woman in a semi-prone position, the partner or doula stands facing the bed and places the woman's upper foot against the partner's hip (Fig. 7.9). During contractions, the partner leans slightly

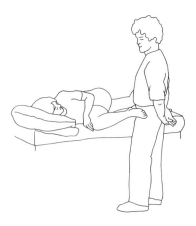

Fig. 7.9 Side-lying lunge.

against the woman's foot to flex her hip and knee more and hold the leg in a more flexed position (Fig. 7.9). It is important that the partner does not lean with all his weight, as it could overstretch the ligaments in the sacroiliac or hip joint and cause later pain and poor function.

What this position does

- Changes the shape of the pelvis, slightly opening the upper sacroiliac joint, and giving more room on the upper side of the pelvis.
- Increases chances of rotation of an OP or asynclitic fetus, is comfortable and effortless for the mother.

When to use the side-lying lunge

- When dilation or descent has slowed.
- If a fetal malposition is suspected.
- When the woman has an epidural and is limited in the positions she can use.
- If the woman is too tired to do the kneeling or standing lunge, and it is desirable to alter pelvic shape.

When not the use the side-lying lunge

- When a gravity advantage is needed to aid descent, especially if second stage progress has slowed.
- When she has been in side-lying for more than an hour without progress.

Semi-sitting

When

During first and second stages.

How

Woman sits with trunk at >45° angle with bed (Fig. 7.10a–d).

7

(a)   (b)

(c)   (d)

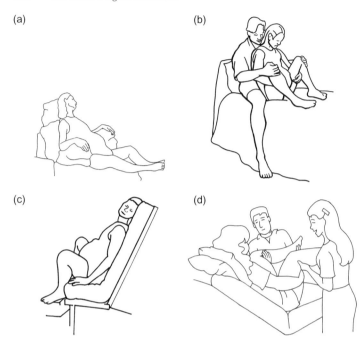

Fig. 7.10 (a) Semi-sitting. (b) Semi-sitting to push. (c) Semi-sitting with bed, back raised. (d) Semi-sitting with people supporting the woman's legs.

What this position does

- Provides some gravity advantage, when compared with supine.
- May be better than supine for:
  - increasing pelvic inlet dimensions
  - improving oxygenation of fetus
- Is an easy position to assume.
- Pressure on sacrum and coccyx may impair enlargement of the pelvic outlet.

When to use semi-sitting positions

- If progress is good, and woman prefers it.
- When the woman needs rest.

- When an epidural is in place.
- For caregiver's convenience during second stage in viewing perineum.

When not to use semi-sitting positions

- With occiput posterior fetus.
- If fetus is in distress.
- If woman has hypertension and this position exacerbates it.
- When the woman refuses, due to increased pain or preference for another position. However, once it is explained that this position might improve labor progress, the woman may be willing to try it.

Sitting upright

When

During first and second stages.

How

Woman sits straight up on bed, chair or stool (Fig. 7.11a–d).

What this position does

- Provides gravity advantage.
- Allows a tired woman to rest, if she is well supported.
- Allows for placement of hot pack on shoulders, low back, or lower abdomen or cold pack to low back.
- Enables woman to rock or sway in rocking chair or on birth ball.

When to use upright sitting positions

- When woman needs to rest.
- When woman has backache.
- When woman finds it comfortable in first or second stage.
- When active labor progress has slowed; sitting up is especially beneficial if her knees are lower than her hips[5–6].

7

(a)

(b)

(c)

(d)

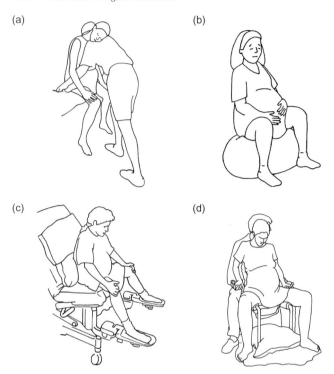

Fig. 7.11 (a) Sitting upright with partner support, in first stage. (b) Sitting upright on a birth ball. (c) Sitting upright to push. (d) Sitting upright on a birthing stool (adapted from photo of the DeBY Birth Support).

- When woman has an epidural or narcotics as an alternative to supine or side-lying.

When not to use upright sitting positions

- When the woman refuses, due to increased pain or a preference for another position. However, if it is explained that there is a chance that this position will improve labor progress, the woman may be willing to try it.
- When fetal heart rate is compromised in that position.

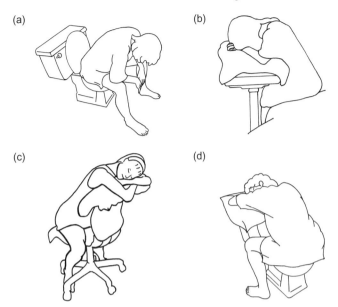

Fig. 7.12 (a) Sitting forward on toilet. (b) Sitting, leaning on tray table. (c) Straddling a chair. (d) Straddling a toilet.

Sitting leaning forward with support

When

During first and second stages.

How

Woman sits with feet firmly placed and leans forward, arms resting on thighs or on a prop in front of her (Fig. 7.12a and b); or she straddles a chair or toilet and rests her upper body on the back (Fig. 7.12c and d).

What this position does

- Provides gravity advantage.
- Is restful if woman is well supported.

7

- Relieves backache.
- May enhance rotation from occiput posterior (when compared with supine, semi-sitting).
- Aligns fetus with pelvis (Fig. 2.2)[7].
- Enlarges pelvic inlet (when compared with supine).
- Allows easy access for backrub.

When to use sitting and leaning forward

- If woman is semi-reclining and labor is not progressing, to shift the weight of the fetal torso off the woman's spine.
- When the woman has backache.
- When woman finds it comfortable in first or second stage.
- When active labor progress has slowed.

When not to use sitting and leaning forward

- When the woman objects, due to increased pain or a preference for another position. However, if it is explained that this position may improve labor progress, the woman may be willing to try it.
- If labor progress does not improve after 6–8 contractions in this position.
- If epidural or narcotics interfere with her ability to maintain this position.

Standing, leaning forward

When

During first and second stage.

How

Woman stands and leans on partner, on a raised bed, over a birth ball placed on the bed, or on a wall rail or counter top (Fig. 7.13a–d).

What this position does

- Provides gravity advantage.
- Enlarges pelvic inlet (when compared with supine or sitting).

(a)   (b)

(c)   (d)

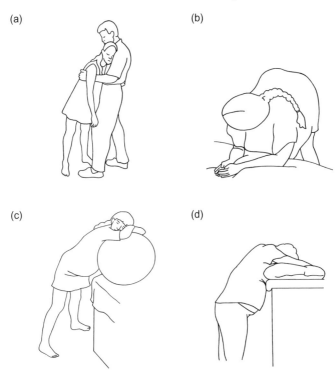

Fig. 7.13   (a) Standing, leaning on partner. (b) Standing, leaning forward on bed. (c) Standing, leaning on birth ball. (d) Standing, leaning on counter.

- Aligns fetus with pelvic inlet (Fig. 2.2)[5-7].
- May promote flexion of fetal head.
- May enhance rotation from OP, especially if combined with swaying movements[5-6].
- Causes contractions to be less painful but more productive than in supine or sitting[1].
- Relieves backache by reducing pressure of the fetal presenting part on the woman's sacrum.
- May be easier to maintain than hands and knees position.
- If the woman is embraced and supported in the upright position

by her partner, the embrace increases her sense of well-being and may reduce catecholamine production.
- May increase her urge to push in second stage.

When to use standing and leaning forward

- When labor progress is slow or arrested.
- When contractions space out or lose intensity.
- When woman has backache.
- When woman finds it comfortable in first or second stage.

When not to use standing and leaning forward

- When the woman objects, due to increased pain or a preference for another position. However, if it is explained that this position may improve labor progress, the woman may be willing to try it.
- When birth is imminent and the attendant does not want to deliver the baby in this position.
- When epidural or narcotics interfere with woman's motor control.

Kneeling, leaning forward with support

When

During first and second stages.

How

Woman kneels on bed or floor, leaning forward onto back of bed, on a chair seat, birth ball, or other support (Fig. 7.14a–d).

What this position does

- Provides some gravity advantage.
- Aligns fetus with pelvic inlet.
- Enlarges pelvic inlet more than side-lying, supine, or sitting.
- Allows easy access for back pressure.
- Relieves strain on hands and wrists when compared with hands and knees.

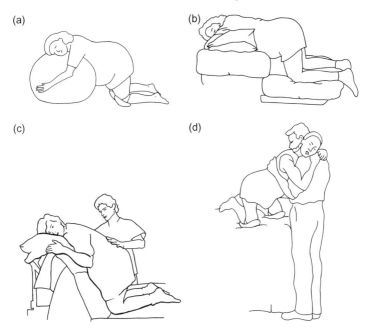

Fig. 7.14 (a) Kneeling, leaning on a ball, with knee pads. (b) Kneeling on foot of bed. (c) Kneeling over back of bed. (d) Kneeling with partner support to push, and knee pads.

- Allows easy movement (swaying, rocking).
- May relieve cord compression.
- May cause soreness in knees (to prevent this, woman can wear kneepads made for sports or gardening).

When to use kneeling and leaning forward

- When fetus is occiput posterior.
- When woman has backache.
- When woman is in a bath or pool, if space allows.
- When fetal distress is noted with supine or side-lying position.
- When fetus is at a high station.
- If woman finds it comfortable.
- To alternate with other positions for backache.

7

When not to use kneeling and leaning forward

- When woman has pain in knees or legs.
- If woman is very tired.
- When first or second stage is not progressing in the position.
- If epidural or narcotics impair her motor control.

Hands and knees

When

During first and second stages.

How

Woman kneels (preferably on a padded surface), leans forward and supports herself on either the palms of her hands or her fists (the latter being more tolerable if she has carpal tunnel syndrome). See Fig. 7.15. Knee pads may make her more comfortable.

What this position does

- Aids fetal rotation from OP.
- May aid in reducing an anterior lip in late first stage.
- Reduces back pain.
- Allows swaying, crawling, or rocking motion to promote rotation and increase comfort.
- Relieves hemorrhoids.
- May resolve fetal heart rate problems, especially if due to cord compression.

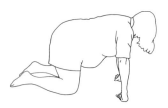

Fig. 7.15 Hands and knees.

- Allows easy access for counter-pressure or double hip squeeze (pages 268–272).
- Allows access for vaginal exams.
- Arms may tire; to relieve, she rests upper body and head on a pile of pillows, chair seat, or birth ball.

When to use hands and knees

- When woman has backache.
- When fetus is occiput posterior.
- When woman finds it comfortable in first or second stage.
- When an anterior lip slows progress.

When not to use hands and knees

- When the woman objects, due to increased pain or a preference for another position. However, if it is explained that this position may improve labor progress, the woman may be willing to try it.
- When epidural or narcotics impairs her motor control.

Open knee–chest position

When

During first and second stages.

How

Woman kneels, leans forward to support weight on her hands, then lowers her chest to the floor, so that her buttocks are higher than her chest. In the open knee–chest position (Fig. 7.16a and b), her hips are less flexed (>90° angle) than in the usual closed knee–chest position (Fig. 7.17). The more open position puts the pelvis at a very different angle from that when the knees are drawn up under her trunk.

7

What this position does

- Protects against fetal distress with prolapsed cord.
- If used for 30–45 minutes during the latent phase or any time

(a)

(b)

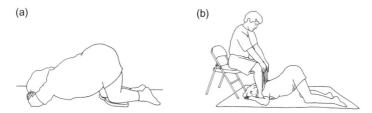

Fig. 7.16 (a) Open knee–chest position with knee pads. (b) Open knee–chest position, shoulders resting on partner's shins.

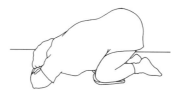

Fig. 7.17 Closed knee–chest position.

before engagement it allows repositioning of the fetal head. Gravity encourages the fetal head to 'back out' of the pelvis and rotate or flex before re-entering.

- May resolve some fetal heart rate problems.
- Reduces back pain.
- Relieves hemorrhoids.
- It is tiring. Pillows and support from the partner makes the position easier.

When to use the open knee–chest position

- If there is a prolapsed cord.
- When one suspects OP in pre-labor or early labor, as indicated by contractions that 'couple', that is, they are are short, frequent, irregular, and painful, especially in the low back, and not accompanied by dilation[8]. This position may be alternated with semi-prone (exaggerated Sims') position. See page 100 for further description.
- When the woman has a backache.

- When it is necessary for the woman to avoid a premature urge to push.
- When the woman has a swollen cervix or anterior lip.
- If caregiver is about to perform a manual rotation of the posterior head during second stage.

When not to use the open knee–chest position

- During a normally progressing second stage (works against gravity).
- If epidural or narcotics interferes with motor control.

Closed knee–chest position

When

During first and second stages.

How

Woman kneels, and leans forward, supporting herself on her hands, then lowers her chest to the bed, with her knees and hips flexed and abducted beneath her abdomen (Fig. 7.17).

What this position does

- Reduces back pain.
- Is less strenuous than hands and knees or 'open' knee–chest position (see pages 212–215).
- Spreads ischia, enlarging pelvic outlet (bispinous and intertuberous diameters).
- Relieves hemorrhoids.
- May resolve some fetal heart rate problems.
- Is an anti-gravity position which may help reduce an anterior lip.

7

When to use the closed knee–chest position

- When woman has a backache.
- When woman has a swollen cervix or anterior lip.
- If there is a prolapsed cord (although open knee–chest may be more effective in moving baby off cord).

When not to use the closed knee–chest position

- In pre-labor or early labor when rotation is desired. (Instead try open knee–chest with hips at >90° angle. See pages 213–215).
- When the woman objects, due to increased pain or a preference for another position. However, if it is explained that this position may improve labor progress, the woman may be willing to try it.
- If the woman becomes short of breath, has gastric upset, or other discomfort.
- During a normally progressing second stage (works against gravity).

Asymmetrical upright (standing, kneeling, sitting) positions

When

During first and second stages.

How

The woman sits, stands, or kneels, with one knee and hip flexed, and foot elevated above the other (Fig. 7.18a–d). Comfort guides the woman in which leg to raise. She should try both sides; one side may be much more comfortable than the other; the more comfortable side is probably the one to use.

What these positions do

- Exert a mild stretch on adductor muscles of the raised thigh, causing some lateral movement of the ischium, thus increasing pelvic outlet diameter.
- May aid rotation from occiput posterior.
- Reduce back pain.
- Provide gravity advantage.
- Allow the woman to 'lunge' in this position, thereby causing the pelvic outlet to widen even more on that side (see page 233).

When to use asymmetrical upright positions

- When woman has backache.
- When active labor progress has slowed.

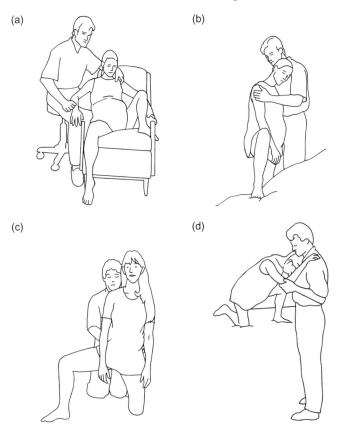

Fig. 7.18 (a) Asymmetrical sitting. (b) Asymmetrical standing. (c) Asymmetrical kneeling. (d) Asymmetrical kneeling with partner support.

- When rotation is desired in first or second stage.
- When fetus is suspected to be asynclitic.

When not to use asymmetrical upright positions

- When the woman finds that these positions increase pain in her knees, hips, or pubic joint.
- When she has an epidural or narcotics that may weaken her legs or impair her balance.

Squatting

When

Primarily during second stage, but any time the mother finds it comfortable.

How

The woman lowers herself from standing into a squatting position with her feet flat on the floor or bed, using her partner, a squatting bar, or other support for balance, if necessary (Fig. 7.19a–c).

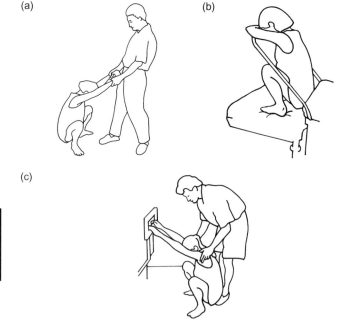

Fig. 7.19 (a) Partner squat. (b) Squatting with a bar. (c) Squatting holding bed rail.

What this position does

- Provides gravity advantage.
- Enlarges pelvic outlet by increasing the intertuberous diameter.
- May require less bearing-down effort than horizontal positions.
- May enhance urge to push.
- May enhance fetal descent.
- May relieve backache.
- Allows freedom to shift weight for comfort.
- Provides mechanical advantage: upper trunk presses on fundus more than in many other positions.
- May impede correction of the angle of the head, if the fetus is at a relatively high station and asynclitic. The pressure of the woman's upper torso on the fundus may reduce the space available for the fetus to 'wriggle' into synclitism. (Positions that lengthen the trunk and relax the pelvic joints may be preferable. See supported squat and dangle, pages 220–222.) However, if the fetal head is engaged and well-aligned in occiput anterior (OA), squatting may hasten descent.
- If continued for a prolonged period, compresses the blood vessels and nerves located behind the knee joint, impairing circulation and possibly causing entrapment neuropathy. As long as the woman sits back or rises to standing after every contraction or two, such problems are avoided. *Please note*: women for whom squatting is a customary resting position do not have these potential nerve and circulation problems.

When to use squatting

- When more space within the pelvis is desired during second stage, especially when fetus is OA.
- When descent is inadequate.

When not to use squatting

- When there is lower extremity joint injury, arthritis, or weakness in legs.
- When it is known that the fetal head has not reached the level of the ischial spines (0 station).
- When an epidural has caused motor or sensory block in legs.

7

Supported squatting positions

When

During second stage.

How

The supported squat: During contractions, the woman leans with her back against her partner, who places his or her forearms under her arms and holds her hands, taking all her weight (Fig. 7.20a). She stands between contractions.

The 'dangle': The partner sits on a high bed or counter, feet supported on chairs or footrests, with thighs spread. The woman stands between partner's legs with her back to her partner, and places her flexed arms over partner's thighs. During the contraction she lowers herself, and her partner grips the sides of her chest with his thighs; her full weight is supported by her arms on his thighs and the grip of his thighs on her upper trunk (Fig. 7.20b). She stands between contractions.

A 'birth sling', suspended from the ceiling, may also be used to support the woman (Fig. 7.20c). The dangle or use of a birth sling is much easier for the partner than the supported squat.

What this position does

- Provides gravity advantage.
- Elongates woman's trunk: may help resolve asynclitism by giving fetus more room to renegotiate angle of head in pelvis.
- Allows more mobility in pelvic joints than in other positions.
- Allows fetal head to 'mold' the woman's pelvis as needed.
- Enables woman to feel safe and supported by partner or sling, which may reduce catecholamines.
- The supported squat requires great strength in the support person, and it is tiring. To make it easier for the partner, he or she may lean back on a wall for support. Make sure he or she maintains a straight back (and does not lean forward at all), and alternate this with other positions. See also pages 222–223.
- If prolonged, may cause paresthesia (numbness, tingling) in woman's hands, from pressure of partner's arms or thighs in her

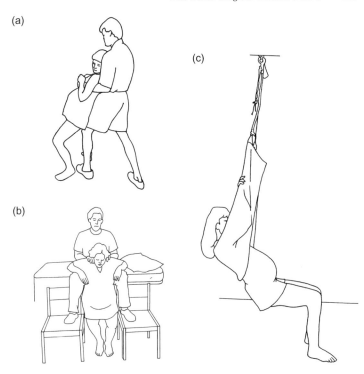

Fig. 7.20 (a) Supported squat. (b) Dangle. (c) Dangle with birth sling.

armpits (causing nerve compression in the brachial plexus). To prevent this, suggest that the woman stands up and leans on her partner between contractions.

- The dangle allows the partner's legs or the birth sling to support all of woman's weight, making it less tiring for the partner than supported squat. (If the partner places his feet directly beneath his knees, the woman's weight is directed straight down from knees through feet, rather than having him rely totally on his muscle strength.)
- The dangle leaves the partner's hands free to stroke or hold the woman.

When to use supported squatting positions

- When more mobility of pelvic joints is needed.
- When lengthening of the woman's trunk seems desirable.
- In second stage, when fetal head is thought to be large, asynclitic, occiput posterior, or occiput transverse.
- When descent is not taking place.

When not to use supported squatting positions

- When the woman objects, due to increased pain or a preference for another position. However, if it is explained that this position may improve labor progress, the woman may be willing to try it.
- When birth is imminent, unless the caregiver has agreed that delivery can take place in this position.
- When the woman has an epidural or narcotics that interfere with her balance or the use of her legs.
- When no one is available who is strong enough to support the woman or there is no birth sling available.

Half squatting, lunging and swaying

When

During first or second stage.

How

The woman stands and, holding onto a supporting device suspended from above (see the birthing rope, Fig. 7.20d), lowers her body and leans back so that she is in a half squat (Fig. 7.20e). She may raise one leg, as in the lunge, described on page 233 (Fig. 7.20f), or sway from side to side, with a feeling of security.

Note: The birthing rope, designed to aid upper body stretching, attaches over a sturdy door, which remains closed during use. The apparatus hangs on the side of the door opposite the direction in which the door opens. The supportive rope enables the woman to maintain positions that would not be possible without it. *Caution*: A support person should remain close by to aid the women with balance.

(d)

(e)

(f)

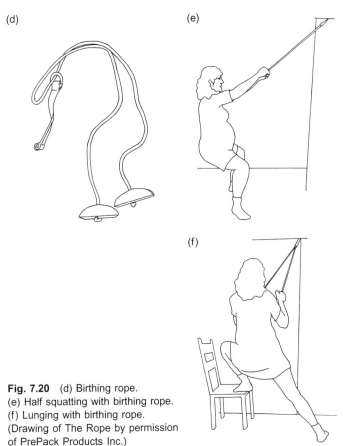

Fig. 7.20 (d) Birthing rope.
(e) Half squatting with birthing rope.
(f) Lunging with birthing rope.
(Drawing of The Rope by permission
of PrePack Products Inc.)

What this position and swaying movements do

- Provide gravity advantage.
- Alter pelvic dimensions when woman goes from standing to half-squatting, and when she sways from side to side in a half-squatting position, or with one leg raised.
- May facilitate fetal rotation and descent.
- May be difficult for the woman to use if she is exhausted or has upper body weakness.

When to use the half squat with lunging or swaying

- When more mobility of pelvic joints is needed.
- When woman is unable to do a full squat.
- When fetal head is thought to be large, asynclitic, occiput posterior, or occiput transverse.
- In second stage, when descent is not taking place.

When not to use the half-squat with lunging or swaying

- If the woman refuses.
- When birth is imminent, unless caregiver agrees that delivery can take place in this position.
- When the woman has an epidural or narcotics that interfere with her balance or the use of her legs.

Lap squatting

When

During second stage.

How

The partner sits on armless straight chair; the woman sits on her partner's lap facing and embracing her partner and straddling her partner's thighs. Her partner embraces her and spreads his or her thighs during contractions, allowing woman's buttocks to sag between. The woman keeps from sagging too far by bending her knees over her partner's thighs. The partner does not lean forward (Fig. 7.21). Another person stands behind the partner. That person and the laboring woman grasp each other's wrists to help support the woman. Between contractions, the partner brings his or her legs together so the woman is sitting on them.

What this position does

- Provides gravity advantage.
- Allows the woman to rest between contractions, if she is held.
- Passively enlarges pelvic outlet.

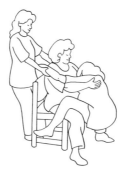

Fig. 7.21 Lap squat, with three people.

- Requires less bearing-down effort than many other positions.
- Relaxes pelvic floor.
- May enhance descent if fetus is occiput anterior.
- Provides mechanical advantage: upper trunk presses on fundus more than in other positions.
- May enhance the woman's sense of security, as she is held closely.
- May be awkward for the caregiver (who must get on floor to view progress).
- May be tiring for the support person who bears woman's weight. The second support person's help in supporting the woman is important.
- May be less effective if fetus is asynclitic or occiput posterior.

When to use lap squatting

- When second stage progress has arrested.
- When woman has joint problems that make squatting impossible.
- When woman is too tired to squat or dangle.
- When all other positions have been tried.
- Can be used with a light epidural. To do this, the woman sits on the side of the bed with her legs dangling and spread apart. The woman's partner sits on a rolling stool and rolls to the edge of the bed, which should be lowered to just above the level of the partner's lap. The partner faces the woman, his or her arms

7

encircle her hips, and the partner slides the woman off the bed onto his or her lap. The woman holds her partner around the neck and her partner holds her around her waist and rolls away from the bed. The second support person (a doula or another knowledgeable person) assists with the transfer of the woman from bed to the partner's lap, and then, standing behind the partner, takes the woman's hands, and the woman and doula hold each others wrists securely. The doula leans back and can easily take much of the woman's weight from the partner. Between contractions the woman sits on the partner's lap and she rests. During contractions, her partner's thighs spread and the woman's buttocks sag between them. Both the partner and the doula hold the woman. At the end of the contraction, the partner brings the thighs together, boosting the woman once again onto his or her lap.

When not to use lap squatting

- When woman finds it impossible or much more painful.
- When there is no strong support person available or woman is too heavy to be supported.
- When the woman has a dense epidural, leaving her with no use of her legs.

Exaggerated lithotomy (McRoberts' position)

When

During second stage.

How

The woman lies flat on her back, legs abducted and knees pulled toward her shoulders (by herself or by two other people, each one drawing one leg up toward one of her shoulders, Fig. 7.22a–c).

What this position does

- May cause supine hypotension, with resulting reduction in oxygen supply to the fetus.
- Is an anti-gravity position.

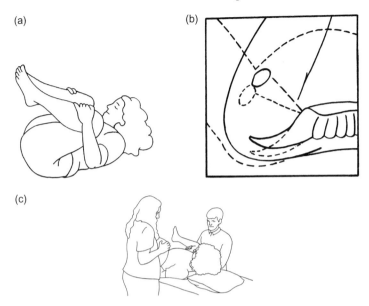

Fig. 7.22 (a) Exaggerated lithotomy (McRoberts' position).
(b) Exaggerated lithotomy (detail). (c) Exaggerated lithotomy (McRoberts')
with people supporting the woman's legs.

- Is awkward and tiring for the woman.
- Puts fetus in an unfavorable drive angle, with exceptions (see below).
- May be beneficial under specific circumstances. If the fetal head is 'stuck' and cannot pass beneath the pubic arch with the woman in other positions, exaggerated lithotomy may help. Pulling the woman's knees toward her shoulders rotates her pelvis posteriorly, flattening the low back and moving her pubic arch toward the woman's head[9–11]. This may allow the fetus to slip under the arch and continue its descent (Fig. 7.22b).

Precaution: If the woman has an epidural, there is danger of injuring her pubic symphysis or sacroiliac joints by forcing her legs back beyond safe limits. Without sensation, the woman cannot feel the joint pain that would otherwise signal impending damage. Those supporting her legs (Fig. 7.22c) should resist the temptation to force her legs back, as they could cause serious long-term damage[10].

7

When to use exaggerated lithotomy

- When gravity positions and positions to enlarge pelvic diameters have been tried, but the fetus remains 'stuck' at the pubis.
- Before forceps or vacuum extraction are used.

When not to use exaggerated lithotomy

- When other, less stressful positions have not been tried first.

Supine

When

During first and second stages.

How

The woman lies flat on her back or with her trunk slightly raised (less than 45°). Her legs may be out straight, bent with her feet flat on the bed, in leg rests, or drawn up and back toward her shoulders (Fig. 7.23a–c).

What this position does

- Allows use of rope pull. (See below for rope pull instructions.)
- Allows easy access for vaginal exams.
- Allows access if instruments are needed for delivery.
- May cause 'supine hypotension' in woman, with resulting reduction in oxygen to the fetus.
- May lead to illusion of cephalo-pelvic disproportion due to the reduced pelvic diameters characteristic of this position (often corrected by changing positions).
- Impedes rotation from occiput posterior or occiput transverse to occiput anterior.
- Requires woman to push against gravity.
- Places fetus in an unfavorable drive angle in relation to pelvis.
- Causes contractions to become more frequent, more painful, but less effective than when the woman is vertical.

7

(a)

(b)

(c)

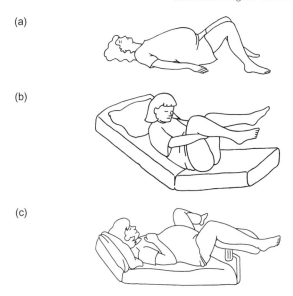

Fig. 7.23 (a) Supine with hips and knees bent. (b) Supine, head of bed somewhat elevated. (c) Supine with leg supports.

When to use the supine position

- When necessary for medical interventions that cannot be done with woman in another position.

When not to use the supine position

- When medical interventions are not needed.

Rope pull

When

During second stage, during contractions.

How

The woman lies flat on her back, with her knees flexed and feet either

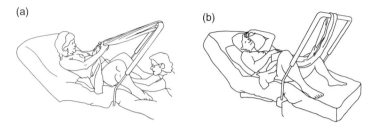

Fig. 7.24 The rope pull. (a) Pulling during contractions. (b) Resting between contractions.

flat on bed or braced on the uprights of the squatting bar. A rope or sheet is looped either around the squatting bar, or around a bar at the foot of the bed, or it may be grasped at one end by a strong nurse, partner, or doula. The other end is held by the woman. When the contraction begins, the woman holds the rope tightly and pulls on it while lifting her head and bearing down (Fig. 7.24a). It is important that she does not pull herself to sitting, but remains quite flat. This maximizes use of her abdominal muscles, which are hardly utilized if she pulls herself to sitting, giving her leverage to bear down effectively. If another person is holding the other end, he or she should brace him- or herself so as not to get pulled over! At the end of the contraction, the woman lies back and rests (Fig. 7.24b).

What this position does

- Aids a woman who may be pushing ineffectively (due to an epidural or some other cause).
- May be advantageous over pushing in other supine positions, but has most of the same disadvantages.
- May cause 'supine hypotension' in woman, with resulting reduction in oxygen to the fetus.
- May lead to illusion of cephalo-pelvic disproportion due to reduced pelvic diameters characteristic of this position.
- Impedes rotation from occiput posterior or occiput transverse to occiput anterior.
- Requires woman to push against gravity.

7

When to use this position

- When the woman is unable to push effectively, especially with an epidural.
- When, because of custom or hospital policy, the woman is restricted to a supine position for pushing.
- When little progress has been made with other positions.

When not to use this position

- When other non-supine positions are possible.
- When the fetus is in distress.
- When supine hypotension is present.

MATERNAL MOVEMENTS

This section contains descriptions of movements by the woman that may:

- Help resolve a fetal malposition such as occiput posterior, persistent occiput transverse, or asynclitism.
- Enhance fetal descent by continually altering the shape and size of the woman's pelvic basin.
- Reduce labor pain, so that the woman is better able to cope with the hours of contractions needed to dilate her cervix and press her fetus through her pelvis.
- Increase the woman's active participation and decrease her emotional distress, contributing to fetal well-being (see pages 265–268).

For information on how to monitor the fetal heart and contractions when women are moving around, see pages 23–30.

7

Pelvic rocking (also called pelvic tilt) and other movements of the pelvis

When

Primarily early first stage, but any time, if desired.

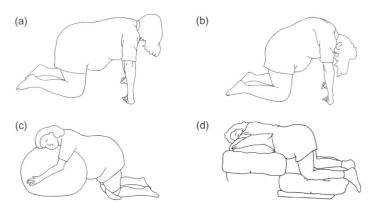

Fig. 7.25   (a) Pelvic rocking, flat back. (b) Pelvic rocking flexed back. (c) Pelvic rocking, resting upper body on ball. (d) Pelvic rocking, resting upper body on birth bed.

How

On hands and knees, the woman 'tucks her seat under' by contracting her abdominal muscles and arching her back, and then relaxes, returning her back to a neutral position as shown in Fig. 7.25a and b. (This is similar to the 'Cat-Cow' exercise used in yoga.) The woman does this movement slowly and rhythmically throughout contractions when she has back pain and presumed OP.

It will be easier on her arms and wrists if she does not bear her weight on her hands but rests her upper body on a support, such as a bean bag, chair, birth ball, or birth bed (Fig. 7.25c and d). Other pelvic movements, such as swaying hips from side to side, are also helpful. The birth ball allows the woman to roll her upper body on the ball: forward and back, side to side, and in circles, almost effortlessly.

Why pelvic rocking helps

If the woman adopts a hands and knees position, gravity encourages rotation of the fetus from OP to OA. The pelvic rocking movement around the fetal head may help to dislodge the head to enable rotation to OA[3,4]. The position and movement reduce back pain, possibly by easing pressure of the fetal occiput on the woman's sacroiliac joint. For many women, this position is the only one they can tolerate when back pain is severe.

Advantages

- Gravity plus movement helps alter the position of the fetus's head within the pelvis, and encourages rotation from OP.
- Relieves back pain.
- If the presumption of OP is in error, this exercise does no harm.

Disadvantages

- The woman's knees may become tired or sore. Knee pads help.
- The belts of the monitor may slip. A support person or caregiver may have to hold the transducer in place (Fig. 2.4) or monitor intermittently. With some monitors it is possible to insert a washcloth between the belt and the transducer (Fig. 2.5) pushing the transducer more snugly against the abdomen to keep it from slipping.

The lunge

When

Primarily first stage, but also second stage if desired.

How

Stabilize a chair so that it will not slide. The woman stands, facing forward with the chair at her side. She raises one foot, places it on the chair seat, and rotates her raised knee and foot to a right angle from the direction in which she is facing (Fig. 7.26a). Keeping her body upright, she shifts her weight sideways (lunges), bending her raised knee, then shifts back to upright. She repeats this throughout several contractions in a row. She should feel a stretch in both inner thighs; if not, she should widen the distance between the foot on the floor and the foot on the chair. Her partner helps her with balance.

7

(a)   (b)

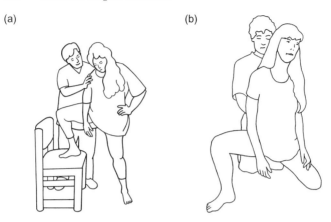

Fig. 7.26 (a) Standing lunge. (b) Kneeling lunge.

The lunge can also be done on a bed in the kneeling position. See Fig. 7.26b.

Deciding which direction to lunge

If the baby is OP, the woman should lunge in the direction of the occiput (e.g. if the fetus is LOP, she lunges to the left). Lunging to this side probably feels better.

Even if the baby is not known to be OP and the woman has no back pain, the lunge may be useful at any time when active labor progress has slowed. The changes in pelvic shape caused by the lunge may correct subtle fetal positional problems. She should try lunging in both directions. The woman will probably find that lunging to one side feels better than the other. The side that feels better is probably the one that gives more room for the occiput to adjust.

Why the lunge helps

The elevated femur acts as a lever at the hip joint, 'prying' one ischium outward. This creates more space in that side of the pelvis for the posterior occiput to rotate, or the asynclitic occiput to resolve its position. Lunging also uses gravity to advantage.

7

Advantages

- Facilitates rotation.
- Reduces back pain.
- Allows the partner to provide physical and emotional support.

Disadvantages

- The woman should have someone (partner, doula or caregiver) close by to help her maintain her balance.
- The woman with joint problems in her legs or hips should not do the lunge.

Walking or stair climbing

(a)   (b)

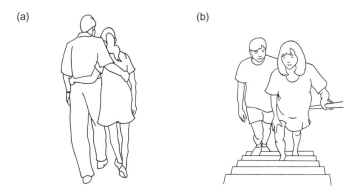

Fig. 7.27 (a) Walking. (b) Stair climbing.

When

Primarily first stage, but also second stage if desired.

7

How

The woman walks (Fig. 7.27a) or climbs stairs (Fig. 7.27b), continuing during contractions if possible. If not, she leans on her partner or the railing. If she spreads her feet wide apart on each stair, in effect she is 'lunging' and climbing stairs at the same time.

Why walking and stair climbing help

Slight but repeated changes in the alignment of pelvic joints occur with each step (more so with stair climbing), encouraging fetal rotation and descent. Walking and stair climbing also use gravity to advantage.

Advantages

- Facilitates fetal rotation.
- Often improves morale, especially if it provides a change of scene.

Disadvantages

- May be tiring.
- Stairs may be inconveniently located.

Slow dancing

When

Primarily first stage, but also second stage, if desired.

How

The woman stands and leans on partner, and sways slowly from side to side. They stand facing each other, with partner embracing woman and pressing on her low back. She leans on him, with her arms relaxed at her sides or with her thumbs hooked into her partner's back pockets or waistband. She rests her head on her partner's shoulder or chest. They can sway to their favorite music and she can breathe in the rhythm of the 'dance' (Fig. 7.28). This is the most relaxing and least tiring way to maintain a standing position, since the woman is partially supported.

Why slow dancing helps

Slight but repeated changes in the pelvic joints occur as she sways, encouraging fetal rotation and descent. The vertical position uses gravity to advantage.

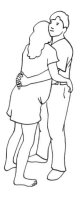

Fig. 7.28 Slow dancing.

Advantages

- Partner's embrace and support may reduce her emotional stress and her catecholamine production, enabling her uterus to work more efficiently.
- The partner provides a kind of support that no one else can give as well. For partners who want to help but feel at a loss to know how, it is most gratifying.
- Rhythmic swaying movements are comforting, and may enable her to relax her trunk and pelvic muscles.
- Partner can press on woman's lower back, providing counterpressure to relieve back pain.
- Can be done beside the bed, with monitors and intravenous lines attached to her body.
- Good substitute for walking.

Disadvantages

- Woman needs a partner with whom she feels comfortable 'slow dancing'.
- Height discrepancies between woman and partner may make slow dancing uncomfortable or impossible.
- Similar physical benefits can be gained if the woman leans and sways over a birth ball placed on a table or birth bed. She can also lean and sway on the bed, counter, or wall.

7

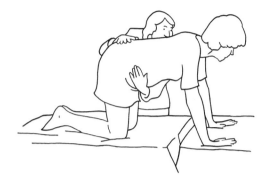

Fig. 7.29   Abdominal stroking for an ROP fetus.

Abdominal stroking

When

Primarily first stage, but also second stage if desired.

How

The woman gets into a hands-and-knees position. Her caregiver or partner stands beside her on the side opposite the fetal occiput. The helper reaches beneath the woman's abdomen and, placing one hand on the woman's side, firmly and smoothly strokes across the woman's abdomen, toward the helper (in the direction toward which the occiput should rotate). For example, if the fetus is ROP, the helper stands on the woman's left side, reaches beneath her abdomen to her right side and strokes her abdomen toward the left. The stroking stops at about the middle of the woman's abdomen. (See Fig. 7.29, Abdominal stroking for an ROP fetus.) The stroking movement is done between contractions, and is rhythmic in character. The stroke should be firm enough to lift the abdomen slightly; this usually feels very good to the woman.

Why abdominal stroking helps

Use abdominal stroking to help turn an OP baby if the position (LOP or ROP) is known. With gravity and external stroking of the abdomen in the direction the baby needs to rotate, the likelihood is increased that the baby will rotate[3].

When to use abdominal stroking

- Whenever the fetus is clearly in an OP position, and the direction of the occiput is known.
- Can be used before labor or during early labor. Success is more likely if the head is unengaged.

When not to use abdominal stroking

- When fetal position is not known.
- When the woman is unable to get into or remain in the hands-and-knees position.

Abdominal lifting

When

Primarily first stage, but also second stage if desired.

How

The woman stands upright. During the contraction she interlocks the fingers of both hands beneath her abdomen and lifts her abdomen upward and inward, while bending her knees to tilt her pelvis[12] (Fig. 7.30a). She maintains the lift throughout the contraction. Her partner (depending on her size and the length of the partner's arms) may be able to assist with abdominal lifting by placing a woven rebozo, or shawl (150–180 cm long, 45 cm or more wide) around the woman, beneath her abdomen, crossing it in the back and lifting her abdomen for her (Fig. 7.30b).

Caution: If the umbilical cord is located low and anterior in the uterus, the abdominal lift might compress the cord. Therefore, it is wise to periodically check the fetal heart tones during a contraction while the abdominal lift is being done. If the heart rate slows, discontinue the abdominal lift. We advise that the abdominal lift should

7

(a)   (b)

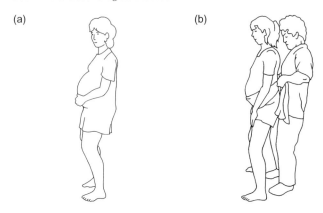

Fig. 7.30   (a) Abdominal lifting. (b) Abdominal lifting with a shawl.

not be done until there is a skilled person available to listen to the fetal heart tones.

Why abdominal lifting helps

Abdominal lifting can help align the long axis of the fetus with the axis of the pelvic inlet. This improves fetal positioning and the efficiency of contractions. Abdominal lifting is particularly helpful for those women with:

- Back pain in labor associated with a fetal occiput posterior position.
- Such maternal conditions as:
  - a pronounced swayback
  - pendulous abdomen (weak abdominal muscles)
  - a short waist (from iliac crests to lowest ribs)
  - some previous low back injuries

Advantages

- Reduces back pain.
- Provides gravity advantage.
- May be done at any stage of labor, from pre-labor into the second stage.

- Sometimes leads to rapid labor (especially in multiparas with pendulous abdomens).

Disadvantages

- Is tiring for the woman if done over a long period.
- Since rapid progress sometimes occurs suddenly, this should not be done with strong active labor contractions until woman is where she intends to give birth.

The pelvic press

When

Second stage.

How

With the woman standing, the partner, caregiver, or preferably two people press her iliac crests very firmly toward each other during contractions (Fig. 7.31a). This should cause some movement in the pelvis, which slightly narrows the upper pelvis. The ilia pivot at the sacroiliac joints, causing the mid-pelvis and the pelvic outlet to widen (Fig. 7.31b). Combining the pelvic press with the squatting position (Fig. 7.31c) may give the greatest chance of increasing space within the pelvis. Within three or four contractions, there should be some evidence of rotation or descent[13-14].

How the pelvic press helps

The pelvic press is a technique for enlarging the mid-pelvic and intertuberous diameters in second stage. The added room may allow rotation and descent in cases of a malposition or 'tight fit' at the pelvic outlet.

7

When to use the pelvic press

- In second stage, when there is a delay in descent or a caput forming (due to malposition or cephalo-pelvic disproportion).
- In second stage, when a woman reports severe back pain.

(a)

(b)

(c)

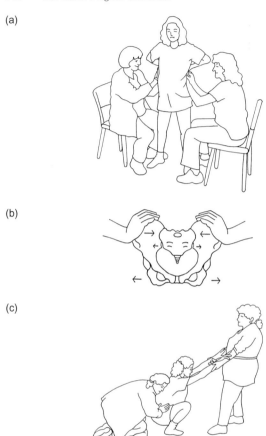

Fig. 7.31   (a) Positioning for pelvic press. (b) Pelvic press (detail).
(c) Pelvic press, woman squatting.

When not to use the pelvic press

- When the pelvic press causes severe bone or joint pain, as it might if the woman has arthritis or a previous injury to her pelvis.
- When the woman has an epidural because, without sensation, joints could be damaged.

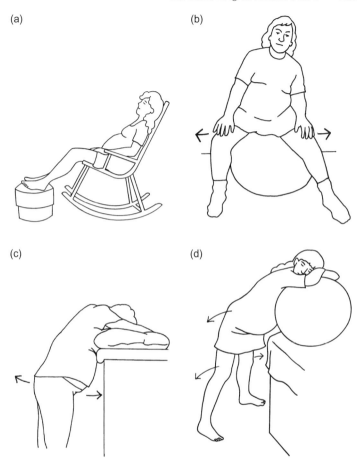

Fig. 7.32 (a) Sitting in a rocking chair. (b) Sitting, swaying on a birth ball. (c) Rocking, leaning on a counter. (d) Standing, swaying with a ball.

7

Other rhythmic movements

When

First or second stage.

How

Moving their bodies rhythmically often seems to occur instinctively in women who are coping well in labor. Rocking in a chair (Fig. 7.32a) or swaying while sitting on a birth ball (Fig. 7.32b) or while standing and leaning over a counter (Fig. 7.32c) or birth ball that is placed on a bed (Fig. 7.32d) are examples of such rhythmic bodily movements. Furthermore, some women find rhythmic stroking or rocking by someone else or by themselves (stroking their own leg or hair, or their partner's arm, or an object) to be soothing. Moaning or self-talk in rhythm is similarly helpful. These behaviors are not planned. They occur spontaneously and instinctively when the woman feels safe. If a woman with slow labor progress is not spontaneously moving as described here, the caregiver might suggest that she try it.

Why rhythmic movements help

- Rhythmic movements tend to be calming.
- Rhythmic movements may alter the relationships among fetus, pelvis, and gravity to promote progress.
- When spontaneous, rocking is often an indication that the woman is coping well.

REFERENCES

1. Simkin, P. & O'Hara, M. (2002) Nonpharmacologic relief of pain during labor: systematic reviews of five methods. *American Journal of Obstetrics and Gynecology*, **186**, S131–S159.
2. Enkin, M., Keirse, M., Neilson, J., *et al.* (2000) *A Guide to Effective Care in Pregnancy and Childbirth*, 3rd edn. Oxford University Press, Oxford.
3. Andrews, C. & Andrews, E. (1983) Nursing, maternal postures, and fetal position. *Nursing Research*, **32** (6), 336–41.
4. Hofmeyr G. & Kulier, R. (2000) Hands/knees posture in late pregnancy or labour for malposition (lateral or posterior) of the presenting part. Cochrane Database Systematic Review; (2);CD001063.
5. Sutton, J. (2001) *Let Birth Be Born Again: Rediscovering and Reclaiming Our Midwifery Heritage*. Birth Concepts, Bedfont, Middlesex, UK.
6. Scott, P. (2003) *Sit Up and Take Notice! Positioning Yourself for a Better Birth*. Great Scott Publications, Tauranga, New Zealand.

7. Fenwick, L. & Simkin, P. (1987) Maternal positioning to prevent or alleviate dystocia in labor. *Clinical Obstetrics and Gynecology*, **30** (1), 83–9.

8. El Halta, V. (1995) Posterior labor: a pain in the back. *Midwifery Today*, **36**, 19–21.

9. Gherman, R., Tramont, J., Muffley, P. & Goodwin, T. (2000) Analysis of McRoberts' maneuver by X-ray pelvimetry. *Obstetrics and Gynecology*, **95**, 43–7.

10. Sweet, B.R. & Tiran, D. (eds) (1997) *Mayes' Midwifery*. Baillière Tindall, London.

11. Health, T. & Gherman, R. (1999) Symphyseal separation, sacroiliac joint dislocation, transient lateral femoral cutaneous neuropathy associated with McRoberts' maneuver. A case report. *Journal of Reproductive Medicine*, **44** (10), 902–904.

12. King, J.M. (1993) *Back Labor No More!!!* Plenary System, Dallas.

13. Koehler, N. (1985) *Artemis Speaks: VBAC Stories and Natural Childbirth Information*. Jerald R. Brown, Occidental, California.

14. Gaskin, I. (2003) *Ina May's Guide to Childbirth*. Bantam Books, New York.

7

Chapter 8

The Labor Progress Toolkit: Part 2. Comfort Measures

General guidelines for comfort during a slow labor, 247
Non-pharmacological physical comfort measures, 248
Heat, 248
Cold, 250
Hydrotherapy, 252
Touch and massage, 257
Acupressure, 259
Acupuncture, 260
Continuous labor support from a doula, nurse, or midwife, 262
Psychosocial comfort measures, 265
Assessing the woman's emotional state, 265
Techniques and devices to reduce back pain, 268
Counter-pressure, 268
The double hip squeeze, 269
The knee press, 272
Cold and heat, 273
Hydrotherapy, 275
Movement, 276
Birth ball, 277
Transcutaneous electrical nerve stimulation (TENS), 278
Intradermal sterile water injections for back pain (ID water blocks), 281
Breathing for relaxation and a sense of mastery, 283
Bearing-down techniques for the second stage, 285
Conclusion, 287
References, 287

Note: Please see Chapters 2 and 7 for general measures to aid labor progress.

In cases of dystocia, there is another important goal besides improving labor progress. That is to help the woman keep her pain within manageable limits, if possible, without interfering with her ability to move freely. This can sometimes be accomplished by using the non-pharmacological pain relief measures described in this section.

We want to acknowledge the benefits of a well-timed epidural in serious cases of dystocia: as a precursor to painful interventions; as an aid for an exhausted mother to get some sleep; and possibly to create, in effect, a 'mind–body split' in cases where deep-seated fear or anxiety is an underlying cause of dystocia. We hope this book will help prevent dystocia from becoming arrested labor, which often necessitates profound pain relief and obstetric interventions for a good outcome.

GENERAL GUIDELINES FOR COMFORT DURING A SLOW LABOR

Following are general comfort guidelines for slow labors:

- Frequent position changes (about every 20–30 minutes when progress is slow) shorten labor, and may reduce the woman's pain significantly. See Chapter 7 for information on specific positions. When progress is adequate, there is no need to change anything.

- Rhythmic movement reduces both pain and anxiety. See pages 231, 243–244 for more information on why movement helps and specific movements to try. For information on monitoring the mobile woman's fetus, see Chapter 2, pages 23–31.

- Pressure techniques, as shown on pages 268–272, reduce back pain.

- Heat and cold, as shown later in this chapter (pages 273–275), reduce various types of pain.

- Hydrotherapy, as shown on pages 252–257, reduces muscle tension, pain, and anxiety dramatically for many women. Immersion in water also provides buoyancy (reducing the effect of gravity on the woman, not on the fetus), even distribution of hydrostatic pressure over the immersed parts of the woman's body, and warmth, often resulting in pain relief and more rapid progress in active labor.

- Techniques such as relaxation, naturalistic breathing and moaning patterns, and bearing-down efforts give many women a sense

8

of mastery over their pain and help them get through a long, potentially worrisome labor. See pages 283–285 for suggestions on the use of such techniques.

- An experienced doula or labor support provider brings to the woman or couple continuous emotional support, physical comfort, non-clinical advice, and assistance in getting information. The use of doulas is increasing, especially in North America, as scientific evidence of their benefit builds[1–2]. In settings where there is a commitment to maintaining normalcy and minimizing unnecessary interventions, doulas and care giving staff have more positive influence than in settings where usual care includes high intervention use and cesarean birth[1–2]. See pages 262–264 for information on continuous support and doula care.

NON-PHARMACOLOGICAL PHYSICAL COMFORT MEASURES

Heat

How

- Apply a hot moist towel, heating pad, heated silica gel pack, heated rice pack or hot water bottle to lower abdomen, groin, thighs, lower back, shoulders, or perineum
- Direct a warm shower on the woman's shoulders, abdomen, or lower back, or suggest she immerse herself in warm water
- Apply warmed blankets to her entire body
- Apply warm compress to augment contractions

How heat helps

Heat (Fig. 8.1) increases local skin temperature, circulation, and tissue metabolism. It reduces muscle spasm and raises the pain threshold[3–4]. Heat also reduces the 'fight or flight' response (as evidenced by trembling and 'goose pimples')[4–5]. Local heat or a warm blanket calms the woman, and also may increase her receptivity to a stroking type of massage which she cannot tolerate when her skin is sensitive or sore due to the fight or flight response.

8

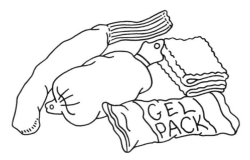

Fig. 8.1 Heat.

Please note: Rice-filled microwaveable packs can be purchased in many department stores. Or they can easily be made by the woman by filling a man's tube sock with 1½ pounds (0.68 kg) of dry uncooked rice and stitching the top of the sock closed. Three to five minutes in a microwave oven set on high, or ten minutes in a covered ceramic dish in a 180°F oven provides moist heat for up to half an hour. Adding lavender seeds or flowers to the rice makes for a lovely aroma. Rice packs can be reheated for the same woman, but should not be reused by other clients.

Caution: If the rice pack is being reheated in a microwave oven, caution should be exercised to avoid contaminating the oven with the woman's body fluids. Place the rice pack in a glass or plastic container or consult your infection control department if this is a concern. (Rice packs can also be frozen to use as cold packs.)

A further caution: Compresses should not be uncomfortably hot to the person applying them. Women in labor may have an altered perception of temperature and may not react to excessive heat even if it is causing a burn. Wrap one or two (or more) layers of toweling, or a plastic disposable bed pad around the source of heat as needed, to ensure it is not too hot. Do not put anything on the woman's skin that feels too hot when placed on your inner arm.

Special cautions on the use of heat with a woman who has an epidural:

- One side effect of epidural analgesia is an alteration in thermo-regulation (an imbalance between the generation of body heat by the contracting uterus and the body's ability to dissipate it),

8

leading to maternal temperature elevation and associated effects on the fetus[6]. If the woman's temperature is elevated, covering her with a warm blanket may further increase her temperature.

- Because a woman with an epidural lacks sensation, never place a hot or warm compress on the area of her body affected by the epidural (even if she reports pain in that area). It may cause a burn.

When to use heat

- When the woman reports or shows pain in a specific area.
- When the woman reports or shows signs of anxiety or muscle tension.
- When the woman reports feeling chilled.
- In the second stage, warm compresses on the perineum enhance relaxation of the pelvic floor and reduce pain.

When not to use heat

- When the woman reports feeling uncomfortably warm or has a fever.
- If staff are worried about potential harm from the heat.

Cold

How

- Apply cold compresses to lower back, or perineum, using an ice bag, frozen gel pack or rice pack, latex glove filled with ice chips, frozen wet washcloth, cold can of soft drink, plastic bottle of frozen water, or another cold object (Fig. 8.2a–c). Figures 8.2b and 8.2c illustrate rolling an ice-filled bottle or cold can of soft drink over the woman's aching back.
- Provide a large strap-on gel pack (available from sports medicine suppliers) to the low back. This allows the woman to move or walk around (Fig. 8.2d).
- Use a cold moist washcloth to cool a sweating woman's face, hands, or arms.
- Place a frozen gel pack or plastic bottle of frozen water against her anus to relieve painful hemorrhoids in second stage.

8

(a)

(b)

(c)

(d)

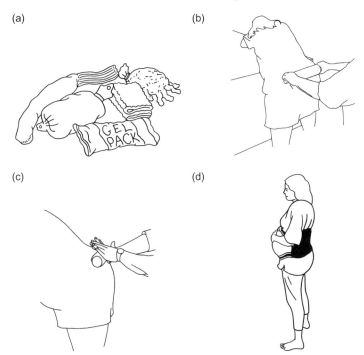

Fig. 8.2 (a) Cold. (b) Rolling cold with ice-filled rolling pin. (c) Rolling cold with chilled soda can. (d) Strap-on cold pack.

Always put one or two layers of fabric or a disposable bed pad between the cold item and the woman's skin. This avoids the sudden discomfort that would occur with the direct application of cold to the skin, and allows for a gradual and well-tolerated shift from feeling cool to feeling cold.

How cold helps

Cold is especially useful for musculoskeletal and joint pain. Cold decreases muscle spasm (for longer than heat). It reduces sensation in the area by lowering tissue temperature, which slows the transmission of pain and other impulses over sensory neurons (explaining the

8

often noted numbing effects of cold). Cold also reduces swelling and is cooling to the skin[4,5,7].

When to use cold

- When woman reports back pain in labor.
- When woman feels overheated, is sweating, or has a fever during labor.
- When hemorrhoids cause excessive pain.
- After the birth, as a cold compress on the woman's perineum to relieve swelling or stitch pain.

When not to use

- When the woman is already feeling chilled. Use heat first in this case.
- When the woman is from a culture in which the use of cold is a threat to the woman's well-being during labor or postpartum. Ask her if she prefers a hot pack or a cold pack or nothing.
- When the woman reports that the use of cold is not helping her or is irritating.
- When the woman has an epidural, do not place a cold pack on the area of her body affected by the epidural. It may damage her skin.

Hydrotherapy

How

Shower: The woman stands or sits on a stool in the shower (Fig. 8.3a and b) and, if possible, she or someone else directs the shower spray where she wants it (on her back or front). A hand-held shower head is more versatile in directing the spray than a fixed shower head.

Bath: She sits, kneels, or reclines in a tub of deep, warm water (Fig. 8.4a–d) with enough space for her to change position and perhaps for the partner to get in.

Caution: Water temperature in the bath should not exceed 98–100°F or 37–37.5°C, because warmer water may raise the woman's temperature and cause fetal tachycardia[8]. The woman should leave the water after $1\frac{1}{2}$ hours or so for half an hour. This ensures the

(a) (b)

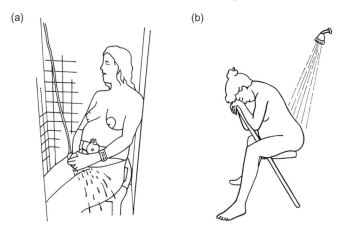

Fig. 8.3 (a) Shower on woman's abdomen (with telemetry). (b) Shower on woman's back.

greatest benefits of the bath. The woman can return to the bath after half an hour or so[2,8].

How hydrotherapy helps

Hydrotherapy (shower or bath) reduces muscle tension, pain and anxiety dramatically for many women.

The effects of immersion in water may be summarized as follows: bathing provides buoyancy and warmth, both of which often bring immediate pain relief, relaxation, lowering of catecholamines, increase in oxytocin, and more rapid active labor progress. The extent of these effects depends on many variables, such as the water depth and temperature, the duration of the bath, cervical dilation on entry, the woman's cultural perceptions, and psychological factors. Benefits seem to be greatest if the water is at shoulder depth and at body temperature, if the woman waits until active labor before entering the bath, and if she remains in the water for a period up to about 1 to 1½ hours. Fluid balance is altered by immersion in deep water. The hydrostatic pressure on the immersed parts of the woman's body (which increases with the depth of the water) presses tissue fluid into the intravascular space[9]. This increases her blood volume, especially in her chest, which triggers the gradual release of

8

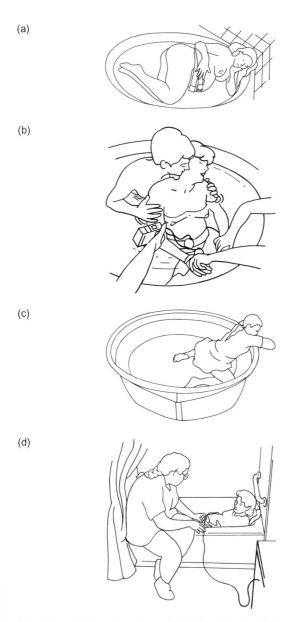

(a)

(b)

(c)

(d)

Fig. 8.4 (a) Side-lying in bath. (b) Sitting in bath. (c) Kneeling in birth pool. (d) Monitoring in bath.

a fluid regulating hormone, ANF (atrial natriuretic hormone). Over time, ANF inhibits functioning of the posterior pituitary gland, including production of vasopressin (another fluid regulating hormone) and oxytocin[8]. Of course, the decrease in oxytocin production leads to slowing of labor. For this reason, women are often asked to leave the bath after 1 to 1$\frac{1}{2}$ hours. They can re-enter the bath after half an hour or so.

How to monitor the fetus in or around water

- Hand-held Doppler device: use models designed for underwater use. If these are not available, the woman must lift her abdomen out of the water or step out of the shower as needed for intermittent monitoring (Fig. 8.4d).

- The older, wired, electronic fetal monitoring tocodynamometers and ultrasound transducers ('belt monitors') are used with telemetry units underwater in some hospitals with women who must be monitored continuously as shown in Fig. 8.4b. These older telemetry units are highly water resistant and because the battery-powered units operate on very low voltage, many hospitals consider them safe for the woman and fetus. The sensors are usually covered with waterproof gloves or long plastic bags. These covers are used more to protect the equipment than the woman[10]. (*Please note*: Before trying this, please contact your hospital's biomedical services or engineering department regarding both safety and any potential equipment damage connected with underwater use of the specific equipment used by your hospital.)

- The newer wireless remote waterproof tocodynamometers and ultrasound sensors can be used for continuous monitoring in the shower or bath. They are attached by belts to the woman's abdomen, but are self-contained and have no wires attached, as shown in Fig. 8.3a and Fig. 8.4a. These cause minimal interference with rest, bathing, or movement by the woman.

When to use hydrotherapy

- As a possible alternative to bedrest for women with pregnancy induced hypertension[9].
- *Showers*: Use in any phase of first stage labor or early second stage.

8

- *Immersion in bath*: Use after active labor is established (with one exception, see below). Because immersion in water often slows contractions if used before active labor[8], a bath is sometimes recommended to stop pre-term contractions or to slow exhausting pre-labor contractions to give the woman some temporary rest. Entrance into the water before 5 cm, however, has been associated with longer labor and greater need for oxytocin augmentation[11]. Barbara Harper, an American expert on water birth, suggests a less strict approach to timing of entry into the bath than awaiting 5 cm dilation, leaving the decision up to the woman. If the labor slows when she is in the water, then she gets out until her labor becomes established, which might occur earlier or later than 5 cm dilation[12].

Note: Immersion in deep water when one is in pre-term labor, pre-labor, or latent labor often stops contractions temporarily through the mechanism described above. This may be desirable if the woman is having pre-term labor contractions, or an exhaustingly long pre-labor; otherwise, it is not desirable because it could suppress early labor progress. If the woman awaits active labor, dilation often speeds up and pain is reduced[8].

When not to use hydrotherapy

Showers

- When the woman's balance or ability to stand is unreliable, due to medication or other reasons.
- When there is a medical contraindication requiring restriction to bed.

Immersion in a bath

- Before active labor is established (unless slowing of labor or temporary cessation of contractions is desired).
- When there is a medical contraindication such as bleeding or fetal distress.
- When birth is imminent (unless woman and practitioner are planning a water birth).
- When the woman has received medications or an epidural for pain.

8

Effectiveness of hydrotherapy during active labor

A recent meta-analysis of randomized controlled trials compared outcomes of immersion in water with no immersion during the first stage of labor. It found significant reductions in epidural use and reported pain in the women who used a bath during labor. There were no differences in operative deliveries, Apgar scores below seven at five minutes, admissions to neonatal intensive care units, or neonatal infection rates[13]. A recent randomized controlled trial found that when dystocia has been diagnosed, bathing significantly decreases the need for labor augmentation with amniotomy and oxytocin[14].

Birth in the water is more controversial than laboring in water, and has strong proponents and opponents. There are few randomized controlled trials of water birth[14], but they are needed to help resolve the controversy.

Showers have not been studied systematically, but clinical experience suggests many women experience enhanced maternal relaxation, and significant reductions in pain.

Touch and massage

How

Various forms of touch, including patting or holding the woman's shoulder or hand, stroking her cheek or hair, even if brief, can convey to the woman a sense of caring, reassurance, understanding, or non-verbal support. Cultural views of this kind of touch vary, especially if it is not given by a family member, close friend, or a female. Women's personal comfort with this kind of touch also varies, so the caregiver must be tactful, ask permission, or observe for signs that the woman wants comforting touch (i.e. reaching for the caregiver's hand, responding positively to a fleeting pat after a clinical procedure). Caregivers also do not always feel comfortable giving this kind of touch and, if not, should not do it.

Massage during labor is formalized touch with the intention of enhancing relaxation and relieving pain[3]. It may involve a specific part of the body, such as the hands, feet, scalp, shoulders or back. It may involve light or firm stroking (Fig. 8.5), kneading, or still pressure. It may include the use of the hands or any of a variety of massage devices. It may be done with or without oils lotions, or powders.

8

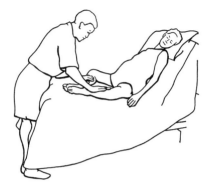

Fig. 8.5   Partner massaging woman's legs.

When to use touch or massage

- When the woman seems tense, frightened or anxious.
- When the woman describes pain in a specific area (i.e. the back, thigh, abdomen).
- When the woman's arms, legs, or feet ache or are tired.
- When the caregiver wants to express empathy, or reassurance.

When not to use touch or massage

- When the caregiver is uncomfortable or unskilled in its use.
- When the woman does not want it, or it is not helping.
- When there are cultural proscriptions against its use.

Effectiveness of touch and massage

One trial of 'reassuring touch' compared with 'usual care' during transition found fewer expressions of anxiety and improved blood pressure in the group who received reassuring touch. Two trials of massage by women's partners, who were taught to give 20–30 minute massages to the women several times during labor, found that the massage groups had less pain and anxiety and reported greater satisfaction with their childbirths than the control groups[3].

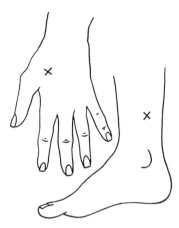

Fig. 8.6 Acupressure points: Ho-ku point on hand (on the back of the hand, where the metacarpal bones of the thumb and the index finger come together); Spleen 6 point on ankle (on the tibia), four finger widths above the medial malleolus (inner ankle bone): apply pressure on the tibia and diagonally forward; this point will be very tender.

Acupressure

How

Pressure on the points illustrated in Fig. 8.6 during labor is thought to enhance contractions without increasing labor pain.

(1) Press firmly with a finger on the point for 10–60 seconds. Then rest for an equal length of time.
(2) Repeat this cycle for up to six cycles. Contractions may speed up during that time. Another technique is to apply an ice-filled washcloth to the Ho-ku point (see Fig. 8.6) on the palm side of one hand and then the other for 20 minutes at a time[15].

How acupressure helps

Acupressure is based on acupuncture theory, which states that specific health problems, including poor progress or excessive pain in labor, arise when there is a blockage of energy flow along particular

8

meridians in the body. By releasing the blockage, harmony and smooth functioning return.

When to use acupressure

- When labor induction is considered necessary. The woman might try self-help measures to start labor, in hopes of avoiding induction, but only after discussing this with her doctor or midwife.
- In labor, when more frequent contractions are desired or needed.
- When contractions are very painful but not accompanied by labor progress.

When not to use acupressure

- During pregnancy before term (unless induction is being planned), because it may result in pre-term labor contractions. We also suggest that the woman should not even experiment with it on herself before labor.
- If she has not consulted her doctor or midwife.

Effectiveness of acupressure

The only controlled trial of acupressure is a study that compared pain ratings before and after ice massage on the Ho-ku point. The women rated their labor pain lower after receiving the ice massage[15].

Otherwise, acupressure has not been subjected to scientific evaluation, so its effectiveness is not certain[16]. However, the techniques are simple and, when used as described above, appear free of harmful effects. They may therefore be worth trying when contractions are excessively painful and labor progress is inadequate.

Acupuncture

How

Fine needles are inserted into the skin at specific points along meridians (channels of energy) in the body. The needles are then rotated, heated, or electrically stimulated. Selection of injection points for labor pain depends on intensity and location of the pain, the stage of labor, and maternal fatigue and tension. Special training, available to mid-wives in Europe, is required. Otherwise, a trained acupuncturist does it; almost always in birth settings outside the hospital[3].

How acupuncture helps

Early descriptive studies and recent randomized controlled trials have reported reduction of pain, less use of analgesics and epidural blocks, and high satisfaction among the women. According to acupuncture theory, as taught in traditional Chinese medicine, the well-chosen application of acupuncture improves energy flow along the meridians and reduces symptoms of pain, anxiety, and poor labor progress. Western medicine does not have a physiological explanation for the action of acupuncture, although this ancient healing approach is being integrated with conventional medicine.

When to use

- When there are skilled personnel available to do it.
- When the woman wishes to use it.
- When labor pain is not being successfully managed without medications.
- When labor progress has slowed or stopped.

When not to use

- When skilled personnel are not available.
- When the woman does not wish to use it.
- When labor pain is being successfully controlled without it.

Caution: Labor may not be the time to educate the woman on acupuncture, especially if a stranger will be brought in to do it.

Effectiveness of acupuncture

Acupuncture for the purpose of augmenting labor progress has not been subjected to scientific trials, but three recent trials found benefit from acupuncture in relieving labor pain. The trials, comparing acupuncture with either no acupuncture of with 'false' acupuncture, found no known risks, lower ratings of pain, or improved relaxation,

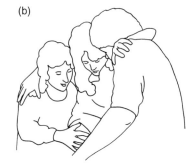

Fig. 8.7   (a) Doula supporting a woman. (b) Doula supporting a couple.

and less need for epidural or pethidine[3]. Acupuncture may be a useful aid for women who want to avoid or postpone, or have no access to epidural analgesia.

At this time, acupuncture during labor is not widely accessible, but is increasingly accepted as an effective option for pain control in labor.

Continuous labor support from a doula, nurse, or midwife

Until recently, and even today, nurses and midwives, along with women's partners, have been designated as the people to provide support to laboring women. Professional staff were expected to add labor support to their long list of other tasks, and it was assumed that any knowledgeable professional could easily do this without instruction. The partner was assumed to be calm and capable enough to 'coach' a woman through labor. But recently, the emergence of the birth doula has shown that effective non-clinical labor support cannot be an 'add-on' to other duties, nor can a loved one provide all the support a woman needs[17-18].

A doula is a person (usually a woman), trained and experienced in childbirth, who accompanies laboring women and their partners throughout labor and birth (Fig. 8.7a and b). She provides continuous emotional support, physical comfort, and non-clinical advice. She is usually a lay person, although some nurses and childbirth educators have become doulas.

8

How the doula helps

The doula focuses on the woman through each contraction, offering reassurance, praise, encouragement, and comfort, as needed and appropriate. She also guides, assists, and reassures the woman's partner. She rarely takes a break and remains with the woman until after the birth. Doulas usually do not work shifts. The doula performs no clinical tasks. Her sole responsibility is the woman's and the partner's emotional well-being and the woman's physical comfort. Some hospitals and health agencies have doulas on staff to help women as they are admitted, but most doulas contract privately with clients. Some work as volunteers; most charge a fee.

In North America, doulas are certified by DONA International (formerly Doulas of North America), the International Childbirth Education Association (ICEA), the Association of Labor Assistants and Childbirth Educators (ALACE), and the Childbirth and Postpartum Professional Association (CAPPA). The concept of the doula is growing in Europe, Australia, and New Zealand. Doula UK represents and supports doulas in the UK.

When to use a doula

A doula should be used whenever one is available and the woman wants her services. There are no known harmful effects when doulas, as described above, are in attendance.

When not to use a doula

A doula should not be used when the woman prefers not to have one.

Effectiveness of doulas

A recent systematic review of 15 randomized controlled trials of continuous labor support included 12,791 women[1]. They found that women who received continuous labor support benefited, but most benefit was found in the trials in which the support provider was *not* a member of the hospital staff with clinical care responsibilities. Care by doulas and other non-clinical personnel resulted in 26% fewer cesareans; 41% fewer instrumental deliveries; 28% less deliveries likely to use any pain medication; and 33% less women likely to be

8

dissatisfied or to rate their birth negatively. Another systematic review of RCTs of continuous support by doulas or nurses in North America found similar results[2]. Support begun in early labor provided greater benefit than if begun in active labor. The women who benefited most were those whose care was provided by doulas as opposed to nurses; whose support was begun during early versus active labor; and those who were not accompanied by a loved one versus those who were accompanied by a loved one.

What about staff nurses and midwives as labor support providers?

'There are two common barriers to be overcome before nurses can provide skilled labor support to their patients: lack of time and lack of knowledge'[19]. While many maternity nurses and midwives enjoy and are skilled in the labor support role, others have little knowledge of these skills, since labor support does not hold a high priority in most educational programs. Even the most knowledgeable and supportive nurse cannot always provide the kind of continuous care that contributes to improved obstetric outcomes, especially if she is responsible for more than one laboring woman or must assume other clinical or 'indirect' patient care tasks that take her out of the woman's room. The largest randomized controlled trial evaluating the effectiveness of nurses as labor support providers included 6915 women who gave birth in 13 different hospitals in the USA and Canada. All the participating hospitals had high rates of medical interventions. The supported group received continuous support from a specially trained nurse who had volunteered to provide the extra support. The control group received 'usual care'. There were very few differences in outcomes between the groups, except for slightly less continuous fetal monitoring, and more indicators of satisfaction with their births at seven weeks postpartum in the supported group. The authors propose that the lack of differences in outcomes between the supported and the usual care groups may be due to the fact that the settings for the trial were highly interventive, relying heavily on continuous electronic monitoring, epidural analgesia, induction and augmentation of labor[20]. The fact that the nurses were hospital employees who were accustomed to functioning within a high intervention setting may also have influenced the lack of differences between the groups' outcomes[1].

What about midwives? Continuous one-to-one care by midwives who focus on psychosocial aspects of childbirth has been shown to produce more favorable outcomes when compared with the usual care by obstetricians[21]. In North America, though numbers of midwives and doulas are increasing, there are still relatively few midwives or doulas. About 10% of births in the USA are attended by midwives[22], fewer in Canada. Less than 5% of births in the USA are attended by doulas. Nurses tend to be very busy with multiple tasks, and must give priority to their clinical responsibilities, all of which leaves many laboring women with little professional support. One can only speculate about the contribution of a lack of emotional support to the incidence of labor dystocia.

PSYCHOSOCIAL COMFORT MEASURES

In Chapter 2 we discussed the importance of a peaceful environment for birth, and showed how outside disturbances may interfere with the labor process. We also described the labor-inhibiting effects of disturbance, fear and anxiety, and how excessive production of stress hormones (catecholamines) can affect uterine and placental function. Chapter 2 also listed some basic and universal guidelines for helping women adapt to the labor environment, and for adapting the labor environment to each woman.

In Chapter 7 and the previous section of this chapter, we provided many physical measures to improve comfort and progress.

This section presents specific psychosocial comfort measures that calm the laboring woman's distress and enhance her feelings of emotional safety.

Assessing the woman's emotional state[23]

It is not always possible to assess a woman's sense of well-being by observation. A woman who is still and quiet during contractions may actually be feeling as though she is 'screaming inside', or 'barely keeping the lid on'. Another woman who is vocal and active may feel okay as long as she can express and release her feelings, or, as one woman said, 'shout down the pain'. A woman's external facade is not always an accurate reflection of how she really feels. Sometimes the best way to assess her well-being is to ask her.

8

To assess the woman's emotional state, it often helps to occasionally ask the woman, between contractions, 'What was going through your mind during that contraction?' Her answer may tell much about her emotional needs, and about whether she is coping well or is distressed. This knowledge will help those around her to provide appropriate emotional support. One important study found that if a woman has distressing thoughts during latent phase contractions (possibly indicating excessive catecholamine production), she is at increased risk for prolonged labor, fetal distress, and all the interventions that accompany such problems. This was not true when women's distressing thoughts occurred in active labor. 'We conclude that latent labor is a critical phase in the psychobiology of labor and that pain and cognitive activity (thoughts) during this phase are important contributions to labor efficiency and obstetric outcome'[24].

Therefore, elimination or reduction of stress is a worthwhile goal, especially in early labor when a woman has little need for clinical care.

The following are specific ways to reduce stress and enhance the woman's emotional well-being.

Provide reassuring or comforting sensory stimuli:

- Music that the woman likes
- Massage, back rub, touch
- Lighting that suits the woman
- Juice or frozen juice bars in a flavor she likes
- Pleasant-smelling hand cream or massage oil
- Making electronic fetal monitoring heart tones audible if the woman finds them reassuring; otherwise, turning them down

Provide reassurance and praise:

- Ask what sensations the woman is having. Explain what causes them and reassure her that these sensations are normal. 'Your body knows just what it's doing'; 'I know this is difficult. It's because you're making good progress. It won't be much longer.'
- Suggest comfort measures to her and her partner.
- Compliment her: 'You're doing so well'; 'Don't change a thing'; 'You're perfect.'
- If she is interested, explain monitor tracings to the woman. Respect her wishes regarding information.

8

- Explain that the vocal woman next door says it helps her cope or push when she yells. And, if culturally appropriate, you might add, 'You might also find that helpful at some point.'
- Help her reframe distressing thoughts, especially in early labor: 'Can you imagine your strong contractions doing exactly what they are supposed to do – open your cervix and bring your baby to you?'

Reduce fear-inducing stimuli and actions:

- Close the woman's door and that of any vocal women.
- Minimize interventions if the woman does not want them (especially painful or invasive ones).
- Ask other staff to make sure they cannot possibly be overheard when discussing their patients. Information and vocabulary that are emotionally neutral to staff members may be frightening to the woman.
- If the woman is accompanied by someone who makes her anxious, ask her privately if she would like that person to leave the room. Send him or her on an errand, or suggest they get a snack. If necessary, ask that person to wait elsewhere.
- Children at birth should be accompanied by their own support people, so the woman and her support person(s) can focus on coping with the labor.
- Avoid bringing unnecessary staff members into the woman's room.
- Provide a more private, less inhibiting environment.
- Remember that nudity or being scantily clad is threatening or embarrassing for some people. Offer an extra gown or robe to cover the woman's back. Some women feel more like themselves if they wear their own clothing in labor, while some want to remove all clothing.
- Keep curtain and/or door closed.
- Knock before entering and encourage other staff to do the same. Sometimes women need privacy, a small space, and freedom from disturbances to adjust psychologically to the demands of labor. Encourage the woman to spend some time in the bathroom with the door closed. Labor progress sometimes improves after some private time. Many women who are 'holding back' during second stage can relax their pelvic floors on the toilet. If you

8

are concerned that the baby may be born suddenly, instruct the woman to push the call light in the bathroom if she feels a lot of pressure.

- Encourage and reinforce the woman's spontaneous coping behaviors, such as rhythmic movements, sounds, and position changes. ('You are good at finding the positions and sounds that work for you.')
- If you are not sure whether a specific behavior is helping the woman or is simply a sign of distress, ask non-judgmentally. ('Does it help to shake your hands during the contraction?')
- Encourage the use of hydrotherapy. Many women 'let go' in the shower or bath.
- If the woman is silent, in her own world, try not to disturb her with questions or procedures.
- If the woman loses rhythm in her movements, breathing or vocalizing, help her get it back, with eye contact, speaking in soothing rhythmic tones, nodding your head or moving your hand rhythmically, so that she can follow the rhythm that you give her (which should mimic closely the rhythm she had).

For ways to support women in pre-labor and latent first stage, see pages 19–20, 92–95. For information on emotional dystocia in active first stage labor, see pages 134–142. See pages 187–192 for information on emotional dystocia and 'holding back' in second stage labor.

TECHNIQUES AND DEVICES TO REDUCE BACK PAIN

Counter-pressure

How

The woman's partner exerts steady pressure throughout the contraction on the woman's sacrum with the heel or fist of one hand (Fig. 8.8). The woman tells the partner where to push (wherever the pain is most intense) and how hard. If needed, the partner places his other hand on the front of the woman's hip (over the anterior superior iliac spine) to help her keep her balance.

(a)   (b)

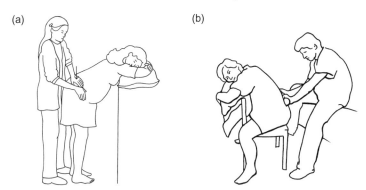

Fig. 8.8 (a) Counter-pressure. (b) Counter-pressure with tennis balls.

How counter-pressure helps

It is not clear exactly how or why counter-pressure eases back pain in labor. It may change the shape of the pelvis enough to ease pain caused by the pressure of the OP baby's occiput on the sacroiliac joints. Judging from its popularity with women, every caregiver should know and be able to teach partners how to do counter-pressure.

When to use counter-pressure

- When the woman reports back pain.

When not to use counter-pressure

- When the woman reports counter-pressure is not helping, or when she finds it distracting.

The double hip squeeze

How

One or two people may do the double hip squeeze. If there is one partner, (Fig. 8.9a and b) he or she places his or her hands on the outsides of the woman's hips, over the woman's gluteal muscles (well below

8

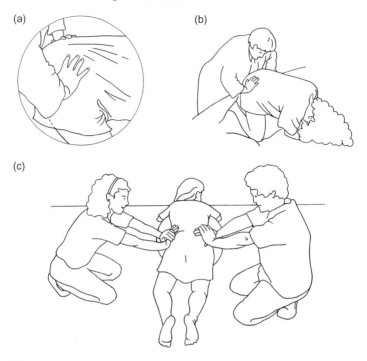

Fig. 8.9   (a) Double hip squeeze (detail). (b) Double hip squeeze. (c) Double hip squeeze with two support people.

her iliac crests, over the 'meatiest' part of her buttocks) and presses inward toward the center of her pelvis with the whole palms of his or her hands (not just the heels of the hands) steadily throughout the contraction. The woman decides how much pressure she needs, and exactly where he should place his hands. This is hard work for the partner. If this is too difficult to continue for as long as the woman needs it, it helps to have another person there to do the two-person double hip squeeze with the partner (see below). If there is no other person to help, then one-handed counter-pressure may be used for a few contractions to allow the partner to have a break. Then he should resume the double hip squeeze if the woman finds it more helpful.

The two-person double hip squeeze. While the woman kneels over a birth ball or the seat of a chair, or, while she kneels on the lowered foot portion of a birthing bed and leans on a pile of pillows placed on the mid-portion of the bed, two people stand on either side of the woman. Each person places one open hand on the side of her hip above and medial to her hip joint. Their other hand covers the first hand. During the contractions, they apply pressure to her hips simultaneously by leaning forward into her hips (Fig. 8.9c). The pressure remains steady through the contraction. They remove their hands and rest between contractions. The two-person double hip squeeze is much easier for those who are doing it.

Note: This is different from the 'pelvic press', which is used in cases of deep transverse arrest, persistent occiput posterior, or in cases of borderline cephalo-pelvic disproportion. See page 241 for a description.

How the double hip squeeze helps

It is not clear how or why the double hip squeeze eases back pain in labor. The pressure may change the shape of the pelvis as does counter-pressure (see preceding section). It may slightly reduce the stretch in the sacroiliac joints, easing the strain on those ligaments caused by internal pressure of the malpositioned fetal head.

Note: The authors consider it a poor prognosis if a woman needs maximum pressure in the double hip squeeze (i.e. requiring all the strength of her partner) in order to get relief. We believe that such extreme measures may indicate that the fetal head is deeply engaged and less likely to rotate spontaneously than when moderate or minor pressure is sufficient to relieve pain. In fact, one may wonder if the extreme pressure would decrease the volume in the pelvic basin and actually impair rotation. This question should be researched: the double hip squeeze seems very effective in relieving pain, but it should not come at the cost of rotation!

Other measures, such as the open knee–chest position (Chapter 7, page 213), abdominal lifting (page 239) the knee press (page 272) or the use of cold or heat (page 273), or the pelvic press in second stage (Chapter 7, page 241), or an epidural may be preferable to maximal pressure in the double hip squeeze.

When to use the double hip squeeze

- When the woman reports back pain.

8

When not to use the double hip squeeze

• When the woman reports that it is not helping.

The knee press

How

If the woman is seated: Woman sits upright on a straight chair with her low back against the back of the chair. She places her feet flat on the floor and her knees a few inches apart. (If her feet do not reach the floor, books or other supports can be placed beneath each foot.)

Her partner or doula kneels on the floor in front of her and cups his hands over her knees. Locking his elbows in close to his trunk, and rising off his haunches, he leans toward the woman throughout each contraction (Fig. 8.10a), allowing his upper body weight to apply pressure on her knees, which is directed from his hands straight back toward her hip joints. She feels a slight release in her low back and relief of back pain. The pressure should be applied and removed gradually.

If the woman is side-lying: with one or two pillows supporting her upper knee, two partners are needed. Only the upper knee is pressed. The woman flexes her upper knee and hip joints to 90° angles. One partner presses on the woman's sacrum during contractions to stabilize her. The other partner cups the woman's top knee in his or her other hand and presses on that knee directly back toward her hip joint (Fig. 8.10b).

How the knee press helps

Pressure directed via the femur straight into the flexed hip joint or joints alters the configuration of the pelvic basin, releasing the sacroiliac joints, and relieving low back pain.

When to use the knee press

• When the woman has back pain.

When not to use the knee press

• When the woman reports the knee press is not reducing her pain.

(a)

(b)

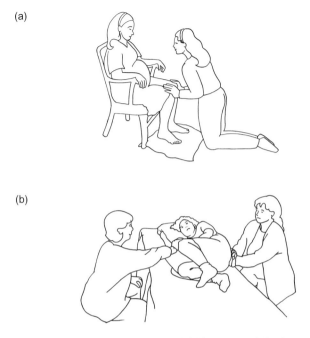

Fig. 8.10 (a) Knee press, seated. (b) Knee press, lateral.

- When the woman has joint pain, inflammation, or damage in her knee joints.

Cold and heat

Cold and rolling cold: See page 273, for the rationale and complete instructions; see also Fig. 8.11a–c.

Note: Always place one or two layers of cloth between the woman's skin and the cold object, to protect her from the sudden shock of a freezing object directly placed on her skin.

Pressing and rolling a cold can of juice or soft drink over the woman's low back is sometimes appreciated more than steady pressure in one area.

8

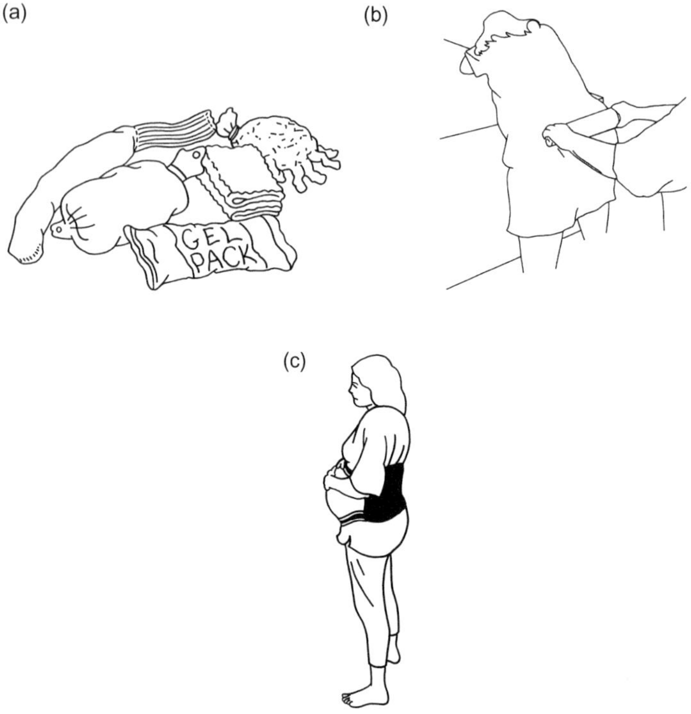

(a)   (b)

(c)

Fig. 8.11 (a) Cold. (b) Rolling cold. (c) Strap-on cold pack.

When to use cold for back pain

- When the woman has musculoskeletal pain (especially low back pain).

When not to use cold for back pain

- If the woman is already chilled.
- If she does not want cold used (for personal or cultural reasons).
- If she prefers heat.
- If the woman has an epidural (cool cloths may be safe).

Hot compresses

See page 273 for more information.

When to Use

- If the woman has low back pain and prefers a hot pack to a cold pack.

When not to use

- If the woman has a fever.

Caution: The woman's temperature sense may be distorted when she is in labor. The cold or hot compress should be wrapped in a towel or pad. Before placing it on the woman's skin, the caregiver should test the temperature of the compress on his or her own inner forearm to be sure the cold or heat is tolerable.

If the woman has received an epidural, do not place a hot or warm compress on any part of her body that is numb.

Hydrotherapy

Note: Hydrotherapy (Fig. 8.12a and b) often results in dramatic pain reduction and may enhance labor progress. See pages 252–267 for instructions on hydrotherapy.

(a)   (b)

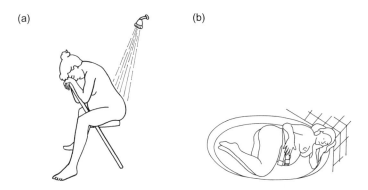

Fig. 8.12   (a) Shower on woman's back. (b) Bath.

8

Movement

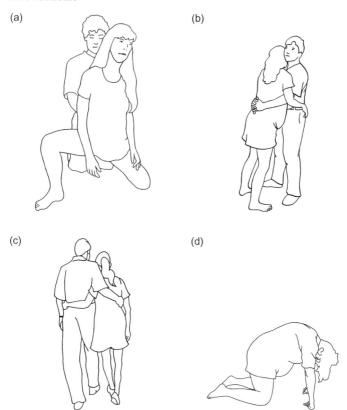

Fig. 8.13   (a) Kneeling lunge. (b) Slow dancing. (c) Walking. (d) Pelvic rocking, back rounded in flexion.

The lunge (page 233), slow dancing (page 236), walking (page 235), pelvic rocking, pelvic tilt (page 231), swaying, rocking (page 244), the open knee–chest (page 213), the abdominal lift (page 239), and abdominal stroking (page 238) all encourage fetal rotation, and some also relieve back pain. See Fig. 8.13a–d.

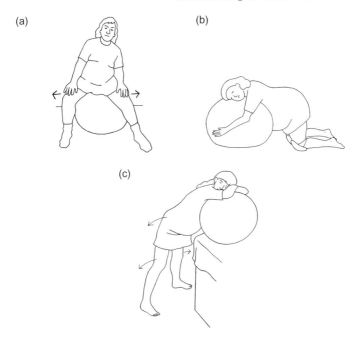

Fig. 8.14 (a) Sitting, swaying on a birth ball. (b) Kneeling on a birth ball, with knee pads. (c) Standing, swaying with ball.

Birth ball

The birth ball (Fig. 8.14a–c) is an excellent aid to movement and relaxation during labor. It is a physical therapy ball. Unlike large balls made for children's use, physical therapy balls are made to support adult weights. Such balls usually have a 300lb (136 kg) weight limit, but you should check with the seller or manufacturer if the information is not included with the ball. The most widely used sizes are the 65 cm and 75 cm diameter balls. For women below 160 cm tall (5 ft. 3 in), a 55 cm ball is a good size; for women between 160 cm and 178 cm (5′3″ and 5′10″), the 65 cm ball is a good size; for women taller than 178 cm, a 75 cm diameter is a better choice. Birth balls can be inflated to varying degrees of firmness and differing diameters, according to the woman's comfort. (Unfortunately, there is wide

8

variation in the actual inflated size of the balls from one manufacturer to another. One manufacturer's 65 cm ball may be much smaller than another manufacturer's. To some extent, this can be corrected by the amount of inflation. Furthermore, the balls do stretch over time and with use.)

The round shape of the ball makes swaying (while sitting on it or leaning over it) almost effortless. It is a wonderful alternative to the hands-and-knees position. Cover the ball with a waterproof bed pad, towel or blanket. The ball can be cleaned with the same disinfectant used on the birthing bed mattress.

Other inflated devices (peanut-shaped or egg-shaped) are available, but they are limited in versatility compared with the ball.

Caution: The first few times a woman sits on the ball, she may feel a bit unsteady. She should hold on to the bed or her partner until she is totally secure. Also, as she sits on the ball, she should hold it to be sure it does not roll away! Once sitting, her feet should be in front of her, about 60–70 cm (2–2½ft) apart. If insecure while sitting on the ball, she can still use it while kneeling or standing. Some childbirth classes provide balls for expectant parents to try before labor.

(Many parents buy balls for their own use in labor and afterwards. The ball is very useful for soothing a fussy baby, when the parent sits on the ball with the baby nestled into his or her shoulder, and bounces gently. This is much easier on the parent's back than walking with the baby.)

Transcutaneous electrical nerve stimulation (TENS)

A TENS unit is a hand-held battery-operated device that causes transmission of mild electrical impulses through the skin, where they stimulate nerve fibers. TENS units (Fig. 8.15a) are available for sale or rent from physical therapy clinics and from medical equipment rental companies, and, in the UK, from many chemists or pharmacists.

How

The four reusable stimulating pads, or electrodes, are placed on the woman's low back on the paraspinal muscles on either side of the spine, two with their top edges at the level of the lowest ribs and two with their bottom edges slightly above the level of the gluteal cleft. TENS units have adjustable parameters that vary with the model used:

(a) (b)

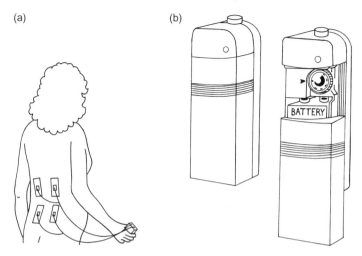

BATTERY

Fig. 8.15 (a) TENS in use. (b) British TENS unit designed for childbirth.

the most common British units, designed for childbirth (Fig. 8.15b), are simple and can be adjusted for intensity and for mode (continuous or burst, off and on). Alternating the mode after a contraction helps keep the woman from habituating to one kind of stimulation, which could diminish its effectiveness. The unit comes with instructions. More complex units, with more adjustable parameters, are also available. These more complex units require the advice and professional guidance of a physical therapist or other knowledgeable professional on how to use it in labor.

The woman or her partner varies the pattern, or mode, of stimulation – 'continuous' mode during contractions and burst mode between, all with a thumb switch. The woman using TENS feels a 'buzzing', prickly or tingling sensation, which seems more intense during contractions and less so between, but always kept below painful levels.

Fetal monitoring: Sometimes the TENS unit interferes with transmission of ultrasound fetal monitor signals. If this is a problem, it can be dealt with by discontinuing the stimulation temporarily so that clear signals are obtained, or discontinuing the monitoring if there is not a medical reason to have continuous fetal monitoring.

8

How TENS helps

TENS stimulates tactile nerve endings, and inhibits awareness of pain, as described in the Gate Control theory of pain[25]. TENS may also increase local endorphin production. It appears to have greater benefit if started early in labor, especially if the woman has back pain.

TENS allows the woman complete mobility, and a sense of control, in that she or her partner controls the use of TENS.

When to use TENS

- TENS is more effective when started in early labor, so it makes sense for the woman to obtain her TENS unit and be instructed in its use before labor begins. Then she can begin using it early in labor before going to the hospital.
- Throughout labor as long as the woman finds it helpful.
- TENS appears to be most beneficial with women who have back pain.

When not to use TENS

- When using hydrotherapy (although she may remove the electrodes while in the water, and replace them when she gets out).
- When woman reports that the TENS is not helping. (She may want to turn it off for a while without removing it. She may discover that the contractions are more painful without it.)
- If there is any irritation of the woman's skin at the sites of the electrodes.

Effectiveness of TENS

A meta-analysis of controlled trials of TENS concluded: 1) there is no compelling evidence that TENS reduces pain; 2) the trials have shown that analgesic medications are used less by TENS users than non-TENS users; and 3) the majority of users would use it again in a future labor[26]. One trial found that TENS users had shorter first stages of labor; used pain medication less often and later in labor, than non-TENS users[27]. Acceptance of TENS by laboring women and their plans to use it in a future labor appear higher than

8

its overall measurable pain-relieving effect[26,28]. Clearly, further study is needed to determine the most effective way (if any) to use TENS, but in the meantime, women's individual preferences should be respected.

Intradermal sterile water injections for back pain (ID water blocks)

Intradermal injections of sterile water are an effective method of reducing back pain[3], and are easily performed by clinical personnel.

How[29]

Equipment: alcohol swabs, and a tuberculin syringe with a 25 gauge needle, filled with 0.5–1.0 ml of sterile water.

(1) Locate the injection sites (Fig. 8.16). The first two injection sites are located over the posterior superior iliac spines (where the 'dimples of Venus' are located). The other two sites are located 2–3 cm below, and 1–2 cm medial to the first two points. A ballpoint pen can be used to mark each site with an 'X'.
(2) After swabbing the site with alcohol, a qualified professional injects 0.1–0.15 ml of sterile water intradermally (not subcutaneously), close to, but not directly on each 'X', to form four small blebs in the skin. The four injections should be performed quickly, to reduce the duration of the pain from the injections.

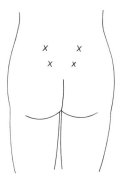

Fig. 8.16 Intradermal sterile water injection sites.

8

(3) The woman will experience intense stinging lasting less than 30 seconds. If the injections are given during a contraction, the stinging is less noticeable. The woman should be told to expect the stinging. Two people can inject the sites simultaneously to speed the procedure, and the woman notices only two instead of four injections.

(4) Within two minutes she will experience relief of back pain, lasting 60–90 minutes. The technique can be repeated.

How ID water blocks help

The mechanism of pain reduction with ID water blocks is not known. Hypotheses include a rapid increase in local endorphin production, or inhibition of awareness of labor pain (as hypothesized in the Gate Control theory of pain). However, 90% of women report significant relief of back pain lasting from 45–90 minutes after receiving an ID water block[2]. This technique has also been used to relieve pain from kidney stones[30].

When to use ID water blocks

● When woman reports back pain and gives informed consent.

When not to use ID water blocks

● When woman refuses.

Effectiveness of intradermal sterile water injections

A systematic review of ID water blocks reported on four randomized controlled trials, comparing ID water blocks with a placebo. All found substantial relief of back pain lasting 1–2 hours[2]. Risks of ID water blocks are the same as with any needle puncture of the skin (minimal when proper technique is used).

A recent study of 60 women's satisfaction with ID water blocks found that 90% were very satisfied or satisfied with the back pain relief, the fact that they could continue to walk around, and the absence of adverse effects on the fetus. The women reported the injections to be briefly and intensely painful, but 71% stated they would use

8

ID water blocks in a future labor; 15% were unsure, and only 13% said they would not use it again[31].

ID water blocks are particularly useful when the woman wishes to avoid or delay pain medications and when epidurals are not readily available (as in out-of-hospital birth settings and some small hospitals). They are simple to give, inexpensive, and safe.

BREATHING FOR RELAXATION AND A SENSE OF MASTERY

Breathing rhythmically, sometimes combined with moaning, seems to be a universal coping ritual during labor. Many women have attended childbirth preparation classes, and have already learned some breathing techniques to use in labor. The caregiver should ask them what they learned and encourage them to use what is already familiar. Many women discover their own unique way of coping, especially in active labor (see The essence of coping, page 135 in Chapter 5). These women do not need instruction. They need support and freedom from disturbance (within the realistic context of clinical care). However, those women who do not know what to do may feel overwhelmed and out of control, anxious, or tense. They can be taught some simple effective breathing patterns, and then assisted in using them during contractions.

Simple breathing rhythms to teach on the spot in labor

How

We recommend that the caregiver be able to teach two breathing patterns: slow and light. These can be taught quickly between contractions.

- *Slow breathing* should be begun at the point in labor when the woman cannot walk or talk through her contractions without pausing over the peaks. Teach her to 'sigh' her way through the contractions with full, easy, audible breaths that may or may not be accompanied by moaning. Combine breathing with imagery. Here are some examples.

8

'Every out breath is a relaxing breath.'

'Send each in-breath to a tense area and breathe the tension away from that area.'

'Imagine that each breath is another step up the mountain, that is, your contraction. When you get to the peak, you can breathe your way down.'

'Let's count your breaths as you go through the contractions. Then (assuming the contractions follow a fairly consistent pattern), we'll be able to tell when you are about halfway through. It will make your contractions seem shorter.'

- *Light breathing* is reserved for a time in active labor when the woman becomes discouraged or finds that the slow breathing is no longer helping very much, even with your encouragement and help. Teach her to breathe more shallowly and more quickly but still at a speed at which she is comfortable through the contractions (for example, one quick light breath every two or three seconds. She pauses briefly after each out-breath to keep from breathing too fast). It is easier for the woman if you pace her with rhythmic hand or head movements, and talk to her soothingly and in the rhythm of her breathing: 'Good . . . that's the way . . . just like that . . . that's right . . . yes . . .' Hyperventilation is unlikely if you pace her and encourage her to keep her inhalations silent and shorter than her exhalations, which should be audible or accompanied by moaning. (If hyperventilation occurs, the woman may need to breathe in and out of her cupped hands, a paper bag or a surgical mask until the symptoms (light-headedness, gulping for air) disappear. Help her slow her breathing down and to maintain a steady rhythm. You can continue the use of guided imagery if she responds well to it. Most women, after being helped with rhythmic breathing through several contractions do not continue to need guidance.

Of course, you will want her to adapt these rhythmic patterns in whatever way suits her best.

(*Note*: If the woman is in advanced labor when she arrives, it may be impossible to teach her very much. If she lacks rhythm in her breathing or moaning, help her find a rhythm by getting her to look at your hand. Move it up and down in rhythm, and say (in the same rhythm), 'Breathe with my hand; that's right; stay with it; good . . .' etc.)

8

How breathing techniques help

Breathing in a consistent rhythmic pattern is self-calming; it encourages tension release and a sense of well-being. This rhythmic self-calming behavior helps to quiet the cortical activity of the brain, putting the woman in a more instinctual state of mind.

When to use breathing techniques

- Whenever the woman seems distressed by her contractions.
- If she has not mastered any techniques for coping with labor pain.

When not to use breathing techniques

- If the woman is successfully using other coping techniques or breathing patterns.
- If she resists trying them, or cannot respond to your teaching.

BEARING-DOWN TECHNIQUES FOR THE SECOND STAGE

Spontaneous pushing

Spontaneous pushing is unplanned and unrehearsed by the woman before birth, and undirected during the birth. Her strong involuntary urge to push usually compels her to bear down effectively in synchrony with strong contractions. See Chapter 6 for a full discussion of the rationale for the various approaches to bearing down in the second stage.

How

When the contraction begins, the woman begins breathing in any way that is satisfying to her, and bears down when she has the reflexive urge, for as long and as forcefully as her urge demands. Each bearing-down effort usually lasts no more than five to seven seconds. The woman may hold her breath, moan, or bellow during contractions, and may breathe quickly for several seconds between bearing-down efforts. This breathing helps ensure adequate fetal oxygenation.

8

Self-directed pushing

Sometimes, due to fear, pain, or 'holding back', women's spontaneous pushing efforts are ineffective, and self-directed pushing is more productive.

How

Self-directed pushing is used when the woman has a spontaneous urge to push but her bearing-down efforts are unfocused, ineffective, and 'diffuse', without apparent progress for 30 minutes. Often her eyes are clenched shut, and she seems afraid or unwilling to bear down into her pelvis.

First, the caregiver encourages the woman to try a new position. (Gravity-enhancing positions tend to help the woman focus her attention.) If that does not help, the caregiver may instruct the woman to open her eyes and direct her gaze and her efforts downward toward her vaginal outlet. Without any further direction, the woman frequently responds impressively, becoming much more effective in her bearing-down efforts. Lastly, the caregiver may have to tell the woman to 'Push through the pain. It hurts less on the other side.'

Directed pushing

How

With 'directed pushing' the woman is instructed precisely as to when, how, and how long to push. She is usually expected to hold her breath and strain for ten or more seconds at a time with only one short breath between bearing-down efforts. This technique is sometimes referred to as the 'purple pushing', which describes the color of her face after a few contractions of this type of pushing.

There are potential risks to this type of pushing. See Chapter 6, pages 150–152, for a discussion of these risks. To reduce the risks, the woman should be directed to hold her breath for no more than five to seven seconds at a time, to take several breaths between bearing-down efforts, and to use a position other than lying on her back.

8

When to use directed pushing

Directed pushing is used if the woman has an epidural, but is best reserved for the time when the fetal head is visible at the vaginal outlet, or the woman feels an urge to push. Directed pushing may also be used if there is a medical problem requiring that the baby be born right away, or if the woman is unable to focus her efforts to push effectively using self-directed pushing.

CONCLUSION

The comfort measures described in this chapter exemplify the nonpharmacological approach to labor pain relief. They reduce pain, while maintaining a sense of mastery and participation by the woman. They make it possible for the woman to utilize the positions and movements described in Chapter 7 to maintain labor progress and, one hopes, reduce the likelihood of a cesarean for dystocia.

REFERENCES

1. Hodnett, E., Gates, S., Hofmeyr, J. & Sakala, C. (2003) Continuous support for women during childbirth. (Cochrane Review) In the Cochrane Library, Issue 3. Update Software, Oxford.
2. Simkin, P. & O'Hara, M. (2002) Nonpharmacologic relief of pain during labor: systematic reviews of five methods. *American Journal of Obstetrics and Gynecology*, **186**, S131–59.
3. Simkin, P. & Bolding, A. (2004) Update on nonpharmacologic approaches to relieve labor pain and prevent suffering. *Journal of Midwifery and Women's Health*, **49**, 489–504.
4. Lehmann, J.F. (1990) *Therapeutic Heat and Cold*, 4th edn. Williams & Wilkins, Baltimore.
5. Nanneman, D. (1991) Thermal modalities: heat and cold. A review of physiologic effects with clinical applications. *American Association of Occupational Health Nurses Journal*, **39**, 70–75.
6. Lieberman, E. & O'Donoghue, C. (2002) Unintended effects of epidural analgesia during labor: a systematic review. *American Journal of Obstetrics and Gynecology*, **186**, S31–68.
7. Enwemeka, C., Allen, C., Avila, P., Bina, J. & Munns, S. (2002) Soft tissue thermodynamics before, during, and after cold therapy. *Medicine and Science in Sports and Exercise*, **34**, 45–50.
8. Odent, M. (1997) Can water immersion stop labor? *Journal of Nurse-Midwifery*, **42**, 414–16.

8

9. Katz, V.L., Ryder, R.M., Cefalo, R.C., Carmichael, S.C. & Goolsby, R. (1990) A comparison of bed rest and immersion for treating the edema of pregnancy. *Obstetrics and Gynecology*, **75** (2), 147–51.

10. Snyder, G., Group Health Cooperative of Puget Sound Biomedical Services (1998) Personal communication.

11. Eriksson, M., Mattsson, L.A. & Ladfors, L. (1997) Early or late bath during the first stage of labour: a randomised study of 200 women. *Midwifery* **13**, 146–8.

12. Harper, B. (1994) *Gentle Birth Choices*. Healing Arts Press, Rochester, Vermont.

13. Cluett, E., Nikodem, V., McCandlish, R. & Burns, E. (2004) Immersion in water in pregnancy, labour and birth. The Cochrane Database of Systematic Reviews, Issue 1. Art. No. CD000111.pub2. DOI:10.1002/14651858.CD000111.pub2.

14. Cluett, E., Pickering, R., Getliffe, K. & Saunders, N. (2004) Randomized controlled trial of labouring in water compared with standard of augmentation of dystocia in first stage of labour. *British Medical Journal*, **328**, 314–20.

15. Waters, B. & Raisler, J. (2003) Ice massage for the reduction of labor pain. *Journal of Midwifery and Women's Health*, **48**, 317–21.

16. Enkin, M., Keirse, M., Neilsen, J., *et al.* (2000) Control of pain in labour, Chapter 34. In: *A Guide to Effective Care in Pregnancy and Childbirth*, 3rd edn. Oxford University Press, Oxford.

17. Klaus, M.H. & Kennell, J.H. (1997) The doula: an essential ingredient of childbirth rediscovered. *Acta Paediatrica*, **86**, 1034–6.

18. Bertsch, T.D., Nagashima-Whalen, L., Dykeman, S., Kennell, J.H. & McGrath, S. (1990) Labor supported by first-time fathers: direct observation with a comparison to experienced doulas. *Journal of Psychosomatic Obstetrics and Gynecology*, **11**, 251–60.

19. Hodnett, E. (1996) Nursing support of the laboring woman. *Journal of Obstetrical, Gynecological and Neonatal Nursing*, **25** (3), 257–64.

20. Hodnett, E., Lowe, N., Hannah, M., *et al.* (2002) Effectiveness of nurses as providers of birth support in North American hospitals: a randomized controlled trial. *Journal of American Medical Association*, **288**, 1373–81.

21. Butler, J., Abrams, B., Parker, J., Roberts, J.M. & Laros, R.K. (1993) Supportive nurse–midwife care is associated with a reduced incidence of cesarean section. *American Journal of Obstetrics Gynecology*, **168**, 1407–13.

22. DeClerq, E., Sakala, C., Corry, M., Applebaum, S. & Risher, P. (2002) *Listening to Mothers: Report of the First National Survey of Women's Childbearing Experiences*. Maternity Center Association and Harris Interactive, Inc. New York.

23. Simkin, P. (2002) Supportive care during labor: a guide for busy nurses. *Journal of Obstetrical, Gynecological and Neonatal Nursing*, **31**, 721–32.

8

24. Wuitchik, M., Bakal, D. & Lipshitz, J. (1989) The clinical significance of pain and cognitive activity in latent labor. *Obstetrics and Gynecology*, **73** (1), 35–42.
25. Melzack, R.D. (1973) *The Puzzle of Pain*. Basic Books, New York.
26. Carroll, D., Tramer, M., McQuay, H., Nye, B. & Moore, A. (1997) Transcutaneous electrical nerve stimulation in labour: a systematic review. *British Journal of Obstetrics and Gynaecology*, **104**, 167–75.
27. Kaplan, B., Rabinerson, D., Luirie, S., Bar, J., Krieser, U. & Neri, A. (1998) Trancutaneous electrical nerve stimulation (TENS) for adjuvant pain-relief during labor and delivery. *International Journal of Gynaecology and Obstetrics*, **60**, 251–5.
28. Wraight, A. (1993) Coping with pain. In: *Pain and its Relief in Childbirth* (eds J.G. Chamberlain, A. Wraight, & P. Steer). Churchill Livingstone, Edinburgh.
29. Reynolds, J.L. (1994) Intracutaneous sterile water for back pain in labor. *Canadian Family Physician*, **40**, 1785–92.
30. Odent, M. (1991) Comments on 'Parturition pain treated by intracutaneous injections of sterile water,' by L. Ader, B. Handsson and G. Wallin (*Pain*, **41** (1990), 133–8). *Pain* **45**, 220.
31. Peart, K., James, W. & Deocampo, J. (2004) *Women's Satisfaction With the Use of Sterile Water Injections for Back Pain in Labor*. University of Ballarat, Horsham, Australia.

Epidural Index

Epidurals, general information about, 91, 125–6, 156–61
advantages of, 107, 113, 122, 140, 247
effects on fetal position, 125–6, 156–9
effects on progress, 14, 106, 125, 156–8, 188
and operative delivery rates, 158–9
variation in degrees of maternal mobility, 158

In first stage labor
and emotional dystocia, 140
if fetus is malpositioned, 125

In second stage labor
care plan, 157
delayed urge to push – options:
    delayed pushing or 'laboring down', 157–9
    adjusting dose, 159–60
    removing time limit, 159–62
    rope pull, 230
    using EFM for biofeedback, 159–61
maternal positions that may be usable with epidurals, 124, 160–1
    if CPD is suspected, 124, 187, 224–5

when the fetus is malpositioned, 166–7, 198–203
    drawbacks of supine, semi-sitting vs. lateral positions with OP fetus, 119
    recommending which side the woman should lie on, 116–17, 167
manual repositioning of fetus by doctor or midwife, 174

Precautions with epidurals
avoiding hydrotherapy, 256
avoiding pelvic press, 242
preventing joint and nerve injuries with lithotomy and semisitting positions, 187, 227
when using cold, 252
when using heat, 249–50

The option of trying other measures first
trying non-pharmacological measures to deal with pain, 125–6
trying non-pharmacological ways to augment contractions (to avoid increased pain associated with synthetic oxytocin regimens), 14, 31–2

Index

3 Rs, (essence of coping in active labor), 135–6, 268
abdomen, pendulous, 15, 97–9, 106, 240–1
abdominal lifting, 99, 113, 120, 176, 239–41, 271
  precautions for, 99, 120, 239–40
abdominal shape, as a sign of OP, 38–9
abdominal stroking, 85, 238–9
abuse, see sexual abuse
active labor,
  definitions, 104
  prolonged, 13
    management of, 105–8
    management styles for, 105–6
    possible causes, 106–11
active management of labor, 13–14, 105
acupressure, 32, 129, 150, 259–60
  avoiding before term, 260
acupuncture, 129, 260–2
ambulation, see walking
American College of Obstetricians and Gynecologists (ACOG), 24
artificial rupture of membranes (AROM), 105, 131
  as a possible factor in dystocia, 88, 111–12
  need for more study, 111–12
  risks, 112
assessments,
  amniotic sac, 55
  caput, 63

cervix, prenatally, 49–50
cervix in labor, 54–6, 122, 150
  see also cervix
contractions, 50, 64–7
  see also contractions
descent,
  abdominal assessment of, 42, 58, 157
  vaginal assessment of, 56–7, 59, 122, 157
dilation, 54, 105, 150
effacement, 54
fetal well-being, 13, 23–31, 50, 69–75, 107, 113, 157, 161
fetal position, prenatally, 37–48
fetal position, in labor, 36, 39–42, 49–53, 60–3, 113, 157, 175
fetal weight, 48–9
flexion, 63
maternal well-being, 50, 67–9, 122, 161
membranes, 55
molding, 63
pelvis, 64
progress in first stage, 75–77, 83, 87–9, 105, 122
progress in second stage, 77, 147
synclitism/asynclitism, 60–2
woman's emotional state, 68–9, 92, 93, 95, 134–6, 138–41, 188–9, 244, 265–6
urge to push, 122
see also emotional dystocia and maternal coping, signs of

asymmetrical dilation, *see* cervical
     lip
asymmetrical positions and
     movements, 118, 166, 176,
     198, 202–3, 216–17
   see also lunge
asynclitism, 15, 22, 95–8, 174–5
   in active labor, 108–9
   and AROM, 111–12
   and cervical lip, 133
   maternal positions for, 97–8,
     177, 203, 217, 220–4,
     224–5, 234
   maternal movement for, 222
   in pre-labor and latent labor,
     95–8
   repositioning *see* manual
     repositioning
   signs of, 60–2, 133
   in second stage, 167–8, 174–7,
     186, 220–1
   see also malposition
augmentation, *see* contractions,
     inadequate

back pain,
   measures to alleviate, 84, 94,
     99, 112–13, 119, 123,
     162–77, 197–8, 200–26,
     231–44, 247–8, 250–4,
     268–83
   in pre-labor and latent labor, 94,
     99
   in active labor, 112–21
   in second stage, 169–73,
     176–7
   as a clue to progress, 76
   as a clue to malposition or CPD,
     111, 123
   TENS for, 94, 113, 173,
     278–80
   see also malposition; occiput
     posterior (OP) *and* occiput
     transverse

bearing down, 149–61, 285–7
   delayed, 156–9
   diffuse, 153–6, 191, 286
   directed, 150–2, 155, 157,
     286–7
   epidural, effect on, 156–61
   epidural, helping women push
     with, 157, 159–61
   fear as an impediment to,
     189–91
   'holding back', 189
   'laboring down', *see* bearing
     down, delayed
   with a malpositioned fetus, 159,
     162–77
     see also malposition, maternal
       positions and movements
       for
   premature urge *see* urge to push
   relaxing the perineum and, 191
   self-directed, 155
   spontaneous, 149, 152–4, 161,
     285
   'trial pushes', 122, 150
   see also Epidural Index; second
       stage *and* Valsalva maneuver
bed rest in late pregnancy, 94
'Belly Mapping', 44–8
birth ball, 19, 21, 25, 85, 97, 112,
     114, 132, 205–6, 208,
     210–11, 213, 232, 237,
     243–4, 271, 277–8
   precautions for, 277–8
birth rope, 222–3
   precautions for, 224
bladder, full, 21
Bishop score, various
     interpretations of, 49
breathing,
   in first stage, 135, 139, 283–5
     when to begin, 90, 283–5
   naturalistic, 152, 189, 249
   in second stage *see also* bearing
     down

supporting and teaching, 20, 268
through contractions in second
    stage, 191

caput, 56–63, 77, 112, 174, 241
cardinal movements, 22, 89
    effect of epidural on, 125, 156
care plan (flow chart),
    anxiety or distress in labor, 139
    delayed pushing with an epidural,
        157
    diffuse pushing without progress,
        155
    'emotional dystocia,' 139
    little or no labor progress, 4
    occiput posterior/asynclitism in
        first stage, 113
      in second stage, 176
    prolonged pre-labor or latent
        phase, 88
    prolonged active phase, 107
    spontaneous bearing down, 154
    urge to push before fully dilated,
        122
catecholamines, 15–18, 92, 134,
        138, 197, 220, 237, 253, 265
cephalopelvic disproportion (CPD),
        13, 15, 22–3, 73, 106, 108
    clues to, 60, 111
    and dorsal positions, 23, 162
    caused or made worse by
        malposition, 106, 108, 110,
        178
    suspected in active labor, 108
      maternal positions for,
        112–15
    suspected in second stage, 177–8
      maternal positions and
        movements for, 177–87
    see also assessments, fetal weight
cervical dystocia, 13, 15, 92, 106
cervical lip, 56, 122, 131–4
    and asynclitism, 133
    interventions for, 132–4, 212–16

manual reduction of, 56, 133–4
    see also dilation, asymmetrical
cervix,
    assessing prenatally, 49–50
    assessing during labor, 54–6,
        122, 150
    difficult to find, 55
    dilation, 54–5
    effacement, 54
    as a factor in dystocia, 15, 92
    position of, 54
    remodeling of, 92
      see also cervix, ripening
    retraction of, 148–9
    rigid os (stenosis), 55
      manual stretching of
        ('massage'), 88
    ripening of, 15, 49, 54, 92
    scarred, 15, 92
    swollen, 55, 132, 214–16
    'zipper' cervix, 55
      manual stretching, 55
cesarean birth, 1, 14–16, 24, 48,
        58, 88, 90, 105, 107, 111,
        113, 125, 127–8, 137, 139,
        176, 178, 190, 192, 248,
        263, 287
cold,
    for hemorrhoids, in second stage,
        252
    for pain relief, 21, 112–13, 172,
        205, 250–2, 271, 273–5
    precautions when using, 251–2,
        273–5
    to reduce swollen cervix, 133
consultation and referral, 12, 73,
        75
continuous support, 248, 262–5
    from doulas, 262–4
    from nurses and midwives, 264–5
contractions,
    assessing, 50, 64–7, 147
    inadequate, 15, 31–2, 106, 111,
        123–31, 188

contractions (*cont'd*)
    and dehydration, 126–7, 188
    and exhaustion, 127, 188
    and immobility, 22, 30–1, 123,
        188
    and medication, 125–6, 188
    and uterine lactic acidosis,
        127–8
  irregular or coupling contraction
        pattern
    as a sign of possible
        malposition, 95, 100, 214
    in pre-labor or latent phase,
        95–101
  non-pharmacological ways to
        stimulate, 14, 31–2
    acupressure, 32, 259–60
    breast stimulation, 32, 107,
        128–9, 150
    heat on fundus, 32, 248
    hydration, 31
    hydrotherapy, 130
    movement and positioning,
        31, 123, 125
    touch, 31
  non-progressing, 67, 83–4,
        104
  patterns in latent and active
        second stage, 147–50
  pre-labor, 93–4
  progressing, 67, 83–4
  tetanic, 129, 149
cooperation between patients and
        caregivers, 3–4, 18–20,
        44–8, 50–3, 92, 137–42,
        190–2
coping with labor pain, *see* maternal
        coping
continuous support by doulas,
        nurses and midwives,
        262–5
cord compression, 73–4, 99, 152,
        174, 199, 211–12
counterpressure, 171, 237, 268–9

cultural factors, 2, 13, 134, 137–8,
        142, 252–3, 257–8, 267,
        274
  non-clinical factors influencing
        care, 7–8, 14

deflexed head and CPD, *see* flexion
        of fetal head on chest
dehydration,
  see hydration and dehydration
'difficult' patients, 136
diffuse pushing *see* bearing down
dilation,
  in active labor, 104–5, 111, 131
  assessing *see* assessments
  asymmetrical, 56, 133–4
  when cervix is scarred, 15, 92
  and definitions of dystocia,
        13–14
  and definitions of labor onset, 83
  when an epidural is given, 14
  and hydrotherapy, 253, 256
  one of many ways to progress in
        labor, 20, 89, 93
  in pre-labor and latent phase, 83,
        87–9, 92–3, 95, 100
  as a sign of active labor, 104
  as a sign of readiness to push,
        146–50
double hip squeeze, 170–1, 269–72
doulas, 5–6, 36, 90, 135, 142, 177,
        248, 262–4
drinking in labor, *see* hydration and
        dehydration
drive angle, 22–3, 227–8
drug-induced rest, 83, 94
dystocia,
  and cesarean rates, 1
  etiologies of,
    cervical, 15, 92, 106
    emotional, 15, 92–3, 106,
        134–43, 188, 189–92
    extrinsic, 2
    fetal, 15, 106, 162–3, 176

iatrogenic, 15, 106, 149, 192
intrinsic, 2
maternal, 106
pelvic, 15, 106
unknown, 3, 108
uterine, 15, 93, 106, 188
    see also contractions,
        inadequate
various definitions of, 13–14,
    82–4, 104–6, 147

early interventions,
    and their place in the care of
        laboring women, 2, 4, 6, 10,
        266
eating in labor, 67, 88, 90, 127
effacement, 76
    assessing, 49, 54
    when cervix is scarred, 15, 92–3
    and definitions of labor onset, 83
    one of many ways to progress in
        labor, 20, 87–9, 93
    in pre-labor and latent phase, 87,
        92
emotional dystocia, 15, 17, 92–3,
    134–43, 188–92
    assessment, 42, 95, 134–7,
        189–90
    common fears, 137–8, 189
    as distinguished from 'holding
        back', 190
    effects on fetus, 17
    physiology of, 16–18, 92
    predisposing factors, 92, 136–7,
        140–1, 190
    preventing, 18–22, 92, 265–8
    ways to help, 92–3, 137–42,
        188–92, 267–8
environment, effect on labor
        progress, 2, 16, 19, 69, 134
    see also emotional dystocia
epidural, *see also* Epidural Index
    adjusting dose in second stage,
        159

advantages of, 107, 113, 122,
    156, 247
avoiding pelvic press with, 242
bearing down with, 156–61
and cesarean rates, 125–6
delayed bearing down, 157–9
effect on fetal position, 125,
    156–9
effect on progress, 14, 106, 125,
    156–8, 189
and malposition, 84, 125, 156,
    200–1, 203–5
precautions when using heat and
    cold, 249–52
protecting woman's joints with,
    187–8, 227
pushing with, 159–61
    see also bearing down
related to various maternal
    positions 200–1, 203–6,
    210, 212–13, 215, 217,
    219, 222, 224–7, 230–1,
    242, 247, 249, 252, 256,
    288
trying other measures first,
    125–6
used more in recent years, 14
exhaustion, 15, 67, 89, 92, 95,
    106–8, 126–8, 151, 188,
    190

'failure to progress', 13, 104, 113
fear, 15, 17–19, 92, 136–8, 141,
    189–91, 197, 247, 265, 267,
    286
fetal ejection reflex, 17–18, 138
fetal influence on labor?, 16
fetal attitude *see* flexion of fetal
    head on chest
fetal monitoring, 23–31, 113, 129,
    176, 189
    audible vs. silent, 266
    auscultation, 24, 27, 36, 43–5,
        69–74, 107

fetal monitoring *(cont'd)*
  brief, when using abdominal
      lifting, 99, 119, 239–40
  comparison with EFM, 70–4
  and cesarean and instrumental
      delivery rates, 24
  continuous, 5, 23–31, 69, 71,
      92
  explaining, 138, 266
  as feedback to aid bearing down
      in second stage, 157,
      159–61
  and hydrotherapy, 27–31, 255
  intermittent, 24, 27–8, 69–72,
      74
  risks, 24
  telemetry, 28, 30–1, 182, 255
  and TENS, 279–80
  without immobilizing the woman,
      22–31, 233, 255
fetus,
  pre-term, 73, 152, 256, 260
  post-term, 73
'fight or flight' response, 17–18, 20,
      248
  using heat to reduce, 248
  see also 'tend and befriend'
      response
flexion of fetal head on chest, 15,
      22, 63, 77, 89, 106, 111,
      168, 174, 178, 209
  after epidural, 156
  effect of maternal dorsal and
      semi-sitting positions, 22–3,
      119

gestational age, 73, 75, 152
gravity, 94, 113, 116–17, 119, 121,
      162, 165, 179–80, 184, 187,
      200–2, 228, 230, 232–3,
      239–40, 244, 247
  as an aid to progress, 5, 22, 85,
      97, 99–100, 110, 167,
      179–80
  -negative ('anti-gravity') positions,
      100, 132, 151, 214–16, 226
  -neutral positions, 132, 197, 199,
      201, 215–16, 219–20
  -positive, 154, 197, 203–5,
      207–8, 210, 216–25, 234,
      236, 240, 286

head compression, 74, 112, 152
heat,
  to augment contractions, 32,
      248–9
  for pain relief, 21, 113, 172,
      247–52, 272–5
  precautions when using, 249–50,
      275
  to reduce 'fight or flight'
      response, 248
hemorrhoids, 199, 201, 212,
      214–15, 250, 252
hopelessness, 92, 93, 95
hydration and dehydration, 15, 21,
      31, 67–8, 90, 106–7, 123,
      126–7, 188
hydrotherapy, 21, 30, 94, 113,
      130–1, 140, 173, 178, 247,
      252–7, 268, 275, 280
  depth of bath, 253
  and fetal monitoring, 27–31, 255
  for labor augmentation, 131
  precautions, 252, 255–6
  timing of, 131, 253, 255–6
  when not to use, 256
hypertension, 94, 123, 201, 205
hypotension, supine, 31, 119, 123,
      152, 186–7, 198, 200, 226,
      228, 230–1

iatrogenic dystocia, 15, 91–2, 106
  see also hydration and
      dehydration; monitoring,
      fetal, continuous; *and*
      positioning, maternal, dorsal,
      problems with

induction of labor, 49, 87–8, 91,
          93, 129, 260, 264
     breast stimulation for, 129
     see also contractions, inadequate
          and oxytocin, synthetic
instrumental deliveries *see* operative
          deliveries
intradermal sterile water injections
          ('I–D water blocks'), 112,
          173, 281–3

labor, normal,
     definitions of, 11–13
          active, 76–7, 147
          latent phase, 76
          second stage, 77
     movement as a component, 12
     psychosocial outcomes of, 12
     work, strenuous, as a component,
          12
     see also dystocia, various
          definitions of
labor onset, various definitions of,
          82–4
latent phase of first stage,
          definitions of, 83
latent phase of second stage,
          147–50
lactic acidosis, uterine, 127–8
Leopold's maneuvers, 40–2
lordosis, lumbar, 106
lunge, 107, 113, 117–18, 170, 176,
          183, 233–5, 276
     instructions, 233–5
     precautions for, 235
     side-lying, 117, 160, 183, 202–3
     see also movements, maternal

macrosomia, 15, 48, 73, 92, 108,
          177–8
     and AROM, 111–12
     see also cephalopelvic
          disproportion (CPD) *and*
          assessing fetal weight

malposition, 13, 15, 36, 73, 106,
          108–12, 177–8
     and AROM, 111
     as a cause of dystocia, 2, 36, 92,
          106–11, 177
     clues to, 36, 100, 111, 133
     and contraction patterns, 100,
          111
     and epidurals, 125, 156–8
     and maternal dorsal positions,
          119, 162, 166, 186, 198,
          227–8
     see also positions, maternal,
          dorsal, problems with
     maternal positions and
          movements for
          in pre-labor and latent phase,
               95–101
          in active labor, 112–22
          in second stage, 156, 162–77
     preventing *see* Optimal Fetal
          Positioning
     see also back pain; occiput
          posterior; occiput transverse
          and asynclitism
manual reduction of a persistent
          cervical lip, 133
manual repositioning or rotation of
          fetal head, 174
     for persistent asynclitism, 177
     for persistent OP, 174
massage, 20, 31, 94, 112, 126,
          139–40, 248, 257–8, 266
maternal coping, 105, 108, 126,
          134, 189, 244, 267–8,
          283–5
     signs of, in first stage, 135–6
          see also 3Rs
     signs of, in second stage, 189,
          244, 266
maternal distress, 15–18
     preventing, 18–21, 68, 92,
          265–8
     see also emotional dystocia

maternal movements, *see*
movements, maternal
maternal positions
see positions, maternal
maternity care practices,
comparison of US/UK/Canada,
8–9
meconium, 69, 72, 73, 75
medication, 15, 51, 72, 106, 123,
125, 139–40
as a possible contraindication to
hydrotherapy, 256
and intensity of contractions, 125
and malposition, 125, 156–8
fewer requests when doulas are
used, 263
and TENS, 280
see also epidural, drug-induced
rest, *and* the Epidural Index
midwifery model of care, 12, 14,
87, 105, 151
moaning *see* vocalization
molding, 15, 89, 112, 174, 178
monitoring, fetal, *see* fetal
monitoring
movements, maternal, 12, 106,
108, 247
as an aid to progress, 21, 22–3,
30, 110, 112–13, 129,
231–44
as a comfort measure, 20–1, 30,
94, 135–6, 231
see also 3Rs of labor coping
effect on oxygen supply to fetus,
22
effect on maternal pelvis, 22,
231–44
and fetal monitoring *see*
monitoring, fetal
specific movements,
abdominal lifting, 99, 120,
176, 239–41
precautions when using, 99,
120, 239–40

abdominal stroking, 85, 113,
238–39
lunge, 107, 113, 117, 170,
176, 183, 233–5
precautions when using,
235
other rhythmic movements,
243–4, 276–8
pelvic press, 169–70, 176,
241–2
precautions for, 242
pelvic rocking, 22, 85, 113,
170, 231–3
slow dancing, 20, 170, 184,
236–7
walking and stair climbing, 30,
123–5, 129, 184, 235–6
see also optimal fetal
positioning

neocortex, influence of, on labor
progress, 16–17
nipple stimulation,
see contractions, inadequate,
non-pharmacological ways
to stimulate

observation, 3, 38–9, 52, 108, 140,
147, 149, 265
occiput posterior (OP), 15, 31, 37,
106
in active labor, 108–10, 113–14
in second stage, 162–77
and AROM, 111–12
and cephalo-pelvic disproportion
(CPD), 106, 178
and cervical lip, 133
determining direction of, 36–48,
109–10, 163, 175
disadvantages or supine and
semi-sitting positions for,
119, 184–6, 205
see also positions, maternal,
dorsal, problems with

increased incidence with
    epidurals, 125, 156–8
and long pre-labor or latent
    phase, 84–6, 92, 95,
    99–100
maternal positions for active
    labor, 31, 112–22
maternal positions for second
    stage, 31, 162–73, 186–7
and premature urge to push,
    120–1
preventing, 45–8, 84–6
re-positioning *see* abdominal
    lifting, abdominal stroking,
    manual repositioning, and
    side-lying positions, 116–17,
    166–7, 198–202
signs of, 36–48, 95, 100, 111
see also back pain; malpositions
    and positions, maternal
occiput transverse (OT), persistent,
    38, 106, 125, 156–8, 178
in active labor, 110
and AROM, 111–12
deep arrest and epidurals, 156
deep arrest and pelvic press,
    169
identifying, 163, 176
    see also assessments, fetal
    position
maternal positions for,
    in active labor, 112–22
    in second stage, 162–86,
    200–2
see also positions, maternal *and*
    rotation
operative deliveries, 24, 58, 98,
    110, 112, 155, 156–8, 159,
    187, 192
Optimal Fetal Positioning, 15, 36,
    47–8, 84–5, 114
oxytocin,
endogenous, 31–2, 129–30, 148,
    158, 253, 255, 258

synthetic, 9, 13–16, 24, 88, 91,
    105–7, 111, 125, 127, 131,
    139, 149, 159, 178, 256
when there is uterine lacic
    acidosis, 127

pain, 15, 21–2, 87, 107, 111–13,
    119, 123, 129, 131, 135–7,
    141
excessive, reasons for, 21–2, 31,
    36, 91–5
as a factor in progress, 2, 112,
    197
patience, 13–15, 53, 56, 68,
    105, 108, 133, 139, 170,
    178
pelvic dystocia, 15, 106, 178
pelvic press, 169–70, 176, 241–2
    precautions when using, 242
pelvic rocking, 22, 85, 113, 170,
    231–3
see also movements, maternal
pelvis,
effect of movement on, 22,
    231–6, 241–4
    see also movements, maternal
effect of position on, 3, 22–3,
    85, 167–9, 199, 203, 216,
    218–20, 227
    see also positions, maternal, dorsal
    positions, problems with
late pregnancy changes in, 22
policies, effect on labor progress,
    2, 6, 21–2, 24, 91–2, 127,
    131
positions, maternal,
as an aid to progress, 22, 84–5,
    94, 97, 99, 176–7, 197–8
categories of, 197–8
    asymmetrical, 166, 198
    dorsal positions, 15, 23, 31
    and drive angle, 22–3
    and instrumental deliveries,
    158

positions, maternal (*cont'd*)
    problems with, 15, 22–3,
        119, 123, 152, 162, 166,
        184–7, 192, 198, 228–31
    forward-leaning, to reposition
    fetus or reduce back pain,
        85–6, 97, 114–15, 165,
        197
        in active labor, 114–15
        in late pregnancy, 85–6
        in pre-labor and latent
            phase, 97–8, 100
        in second stage, 164–5
    gravity negative ('anti-gravity'),
        100, 132, 151, 214–16
    gravity neutral, 132, 197, 199,
        201, 215–16, 219–20
    gravity positive, 154, 197,
        203–5, 207–8, 210, 216–25,
        228, 236, 284, 286
    horizontal, 30, 125, 150, 192,
        219
    for tired women, 128
    specific positions:
    asymmetrical, 198
        asymmetrical upright, 166,
            176, 216–17
        asymetrical horizontal *see*
            side-lying lunge
    dangle and birth sling, 167–9,
        176–7, 180, 219–21, 225
    exaggerated lithotomy
        (McRoberts') use of, 186–8,
        198, 226–8
        precautions for, 187, 227
    hands and knees, 113–14,
        121–2, 132, 212–13, 238,
        276
    knee–chest positions,
        open, 85, 100–1, 113–14,
            121–2, 132, 176, 213–15,
            276
            and hemorrhoids, 214
        closed, 100–1, 215–16
    kneeling leaning forward with
        support, 85, 112, 114–15,
        118, 121, 128, 132,
        210–12
    rollover sequence, 123–4
    rope pull, 229–31
    semi-sitting, 97–8, 119,
        123–4, 203–5
    side-lying, (lateral and
        semi-prone), 85, 116–17,
        123–4, 128, 133, 166,
        198–203
        which side to lie on if fetus
            is malpositioned, 116–17,
            200–1
    side-lying lunge, 117, 160,
        183, 202–3
    sitting,
        leaning forward, 86,
            115, 128, 130,
            207–8
        upright, 179, 205–7
    squatting positions, 150, 153,
        158, 160, 165–8, 177,
        180–1, 218–26
        half-squatting, 222–4
            precautions for, 222
        lap squatting, 224–6
            precautions for, 226
        supported squatting, 220–2
            precautions for, 222
    standing leaning forward, 85,
        98, 115, 208–10
    supine, 5, 23, 119, 123,
        185–7, 228–9
    see also dorsal positions,
        problems with
    Why focus on maternal position?
        22
post-traumatic stress disorder
        (PTSD), 18, 53
pre-labor and latent phase,
    prolonged, 87, 91–3
    definitions of, 83

'false' labor, 83–4, 93
general suggestions for, 93–5,
    214–16, 240, 256
    see also contractions, irregular
        or coupling
management styles for, 83, 87
'over-reacting' to labor, 91
possible causes, 15, 87–8,
    91–3
premature rupture of the
    membranes (PROM) 111
previous back injury, 99
previous trauma, effect on labor
    progress *see* emotional
    dystocia
psychosocial comfort measures,
    16–20, 265–8
    see also emotional dystocia *and*
        vaginal exams, instructions
        for
pushing *see* bearing down
'pushing postons' as distinguished
    from 'delivery positions',
    165

relaxation, 19–20, 22, 90, 94, 130,
    135–6, 142, 191–2, 197,
    247, 250, 253, 257, 261,
    277, 283
    as one of 3Rs, 135, 268
respect, 16, 19–20, 139–41, 266
restriction to bed, 24, 92, 94, 106,
    158, 256
rhythm, 20–1, 132, 236–8, 244,
    247, 268, 283–5
    as one of 3Rs, 135, 268
ritual, as one of 3Rs, 135–6, 283
rollover sequence, 123–4
rope pull, 229–31
rotation, 22, 51, 60, 77, 84, 89,
    100, 105, 110, 112, 113,
    117–119
    encouraging in pre- and early
        labor, 84–5, 100–1

after an epidural, 125, 156–9
after AROM with a
    malpositioned fetus, 111–12
in latent phase of second stage,
    149
positions to encourage, 112–20,
    162–74
    see also movements, maternal
        and positions, maternal
six ways to progress in labor, 20,
    87–9, 93
Royal College of Obstetricians and
    Gynaecologists, 24

second stage,
    definition of, 146
    epidural during, 156–61
    fear as an impediment to
        progress, 188–92
    management styles for, 146–7,
        150–62
    phases of, 147–51
    positions for,
        see positions, maternal
    prolonged latent phase of, 150
    prolonged, possible causes, 162,
        188
    pushing during latent phase,
        149–50
    time limits on, 159, 161–2
    Valsalva maneuver during,
        150–2
    see also bearing down
sexual abuse survivors,
    vaginal exam with, 53
    needs of, during labor, 92,
        140–1, 190
short waist, 99, 106
    see also abdominal lifting
shoulder dystocia, 188
six ways to progress in labor, 20,
    87–9, 93
slow dancing, 20, 25, 170, 184,
    236–7, 276

Society of Obstetricians and
        Gynecologists of Canada
        (SOGC), 24
station, assessing,
  see assessments, descent
supine positions *see* positions,
        maternal, dorsal positions
survivors of abuse, *see* abuse,
        survivors of

'tend and befriend' response, 17–18
time as an ally, 3, 178
touch and massage, 20, 94, 257
  and endogenous oxytocin
        production, 31, 258
transcutaneous electrical nerve
        stimulation (TENS) for
        back pain, 94, 112, 173,
        278–81
  not for use during hydrotherapy,
        280
trial and error, 3, 13, 108, 162
trust, ways to enhance, 16–21, 91,
        125, 137–42, 266–8

UK/US/Canada, differences in
        maternity care, 8–9
ultrasound predictions of fetal size,
        48–9, 108, 178
ultrasound to identify fetal position,
        42–3, 45, 56, 62
urge to push, 147, 153–4, 189,
        190, 285–7
  absence of, during latent phase
        of second stage, 147–50,
        154
  bearing down with, 147
  delayed, reasons for, 148–9
  and epidural anesthesia, 156–9
    see also Epidural Index

premature
  as a sign of possible
        malposition or CPD, 111,
        120–2
  ways to deal with, 120–2,
        214–15
  ways to enhance, 150, 210, 219
    see also second stage, latent
        phase of
uterine dystocia, 15, 123–31
    see also contractions,
        inadequate

vaginal birth after cesarean
        (VBAC), 137, 190
vaginal exams,
  and sexual abuse survivors, 140–1
  fear of, 53, 140–1
  indications for, 51, 157
  instructions for, 51–7, 59–64
  reactions to, in early labor, 91
  timing of, 51, 150
  with various maternal positions,
        52
    see also assessments
Valsalva maneuver,
  history of prescribing, 151
  problems caused by, 149–52,
        156
  alternatives, when women have
        epidurals, 159–61
visualization, 94, 139–40
vocalization, 20, 94, 135–6, 285

walking and stair climbing *see*
        movements, maternal
woman as key to solution in
        problem labors, 3
World Health Organization (WHO),
        2, 11–12, 57